Redefin

Your

W

MIND BODY FOOD

MADISON MADDEN, A.D.

MIND BODY FOOD

Quantity sales special discounts are available on quantity purchases by corporations, associations, and others. For details, contact the publisher at the address above.

Orders by U.S. and Canada trade bookstores and wholesalers. Email info@ BeyondPublishing.net

The Beyond Publishing Speakers Bureau can bring authors to your live event. For more information or to book an event contact the Beyond Publishing Speakers Bureau speak@BeyondPublishing.net

The Author can be reached directly at info@BeyondPublishing.net

Manufactured and printed in the United States of America distributed globally by BeyondPublishing.net

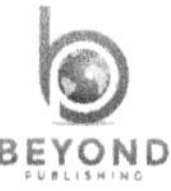

New York | Los Angeles | London | Sydney

ISBN Hardcover: 978-1-63792-190-6

ISBN Softcover: 978-1-63792-188-3

TABLE OF CONTENTS

／
ACKNOWLEDGEMENTS

To all of the people who helped make this book a reality – Your support and enthusiasm mean the world to me.

Thank you:

Colin, for your kind, committed encouragement to bring this to life.

Rocco for taking on the cover design like it was your own.

My teachers and mentors who have embraced and lit the path for me, namely –

Joe Rich, Mamta Landerman, Peggy Berg, Dr. Suhas & Manisha Kshirsagar, Dr. Jayarajan Kodikannath, Dr. Avinash & Bharati Lele, and Dr. Nandan Lele.

To the lineage of Ayurvedic Vaidyas who have passed down the invaluable knowledge of Ayurveda, the *Science of Life,* for more than 5000 years.

To all of the healers and doctors who supported me in learning to heal myself.

To all of my clients who have entrusted me in helping them do the same, especially those whose stories are used here.

… and thank you to the readers to come who invite a new perspective into their life. May it serve you in your journey towards well-being, a journey that is inherently inward.

Dedicated to Ji, who taught me that food is good

And so much more.

FORWARD

"Mind Body Food: Redefining Your Relationship to Food" is an excellent manual to understanding that what you eat and digest is exactly who you become. Food is information and it unleashes a complex cascade of information to every cell and gene which dictates your entire physiology.

Ayurveda is one of the most ancient and comprehensive sciences of healthcare. It's accurate translation, the science of life, gives us the wisdom to understand the impact of our life experiences on health and disease. The rich tradition of Ayurvedic medicine has existed for thousands of years and modern medical research is finally catching up with the vast and vibrant understanding of its medical philosophy.

"Mind Body Food" is a cornerstone for optimum well-being that allows you to develop a spiritual attitude towards life.

I have known Madison Madden for many years. She is a passionate Ayurvedic Practitioner who not only understands and teaches the principles of Ayurveda but also leads a pure, holistic lifestyle herself. This book is a true testimony of her commitment towards the education and daily practice of Self Care Rituals.

We are currently living in unprecedented times. The pandemic, global warming, and industrialization of food is posing a great threat to the survival of the human race.

We are surrounded with food that is filled with chemicals, artificial colors, additives, and toxins. These foods are not only adversely affecting our cells and tissues but also creating a detrimental impact on our minds.

As a global community we are becoming impatient, restless, and hostile. We are creating loads of NCDs (Non-Communicable Diseases) which are the direct by-products of poor nutrition.

We are facing a silent epidemic of inflammation that is triggered by unhealthy foods, weak digestion, and poor emotional health.

My book, "The Hot Belly Diet" published in 2015 highlights the importance of clean foods and a robust digestion. During my research I found that "eating late" and "sleeping late" were the main causes of weight gain, low energy, and a host of metabolic disorders. The punchline here is to eat less, eat right, and become bright. If you rekindle your agni (that is, digestive fire) you can invariably rekindle your life!

The very premise of my recent book published in 2018, "Change Your Schedule, Change Your Life" states that "Time" is deeply embedded in our genes. The old adage "you are what you eat" no longer holds true. It is all about aligning your daily routine with Circadian Rhythms. You also are when you eat, when you sleep, and when you exercise.

The new advances of Nutri-Genomics make it very clear that your genes express whatever you desire. You can turn your genes on or off with your thoughts, feelings, and emotions. Ayurveda stipulates that health is in fact a by-product of enlightenment. You need to be spiritually evolved to deal with the polarities of mind and body. The mind-body system is like a feedback loop where your self-care or self-neglect will affect your lifestyle, inner and outer environment, behavior, past conditioning, and beliefs – and vice versa!

"Mind Body Food" talks about emotional eating, restorative food practices and nurturing yourself not only with food but with every sensory experience.

I welcome you on this wonderful journey with Madison Madden in exploring Ayurvedic medicine.

She has a unique way of translating ancient wisdom for a modern audience. She lives an ayurvedic lifestyle and shows her readers how to apply these practical principles to their daily living. This is a great start for you to find your own path to Health and Wholeness.

Dr. Suhas Kshirsagar BAMS MD(Ayurveda)

Best Selling Author: "The Hot Belly Diet" & "Change Your Schedule Change Your Life"

PREFACE

You have been *seeing* food longer than any other intimate relationship in your life. Whether you like it or not, you have been engaging in an intimate exchange with food from the moment you were conceived and will be until the day you die.

You've probably got a love-hate relationship, some codependent dynamics, and likely patterns of poor communication.

Unlike other partnerships, however, you really *can't* break up with it.

Sometimes your relationship feels comforting, sometimes destructive, sometimes obsessive, and other times appalling. Sometimes it feels rewarding, while other times it's riddled with punishment. You may feel guilt or shame when you relate to it, and it often triggers your childhood traumas.

Sometimes it feels like a never-ending battle for control, in which sometimes you're winning, and other times you're not.

You even experience your sensual and erotic nature with it. You fantasize about it. You think about what your family and friends think about your relationship. You even start or end other relationships based on your views and experiences of it.

You wonder if it will really always be there for you and question what's really inside of it.

Wouldn't it be nice to strike a great balance between knowing it's always there to feed you, and that there is still some mystery, novelty, and rebellion in the mix? Kind of like a partner with whom you have a loving committed relationship, but who can also provide really great sex when you're in the mood...

If you were to describe your relationship with food like you would an intimate relationship with a romantic partner, how would you describe it?

A few years ago, my relationship with food would have sounded something like this:

> *We have an insecure bond. From early on, I wasn't always sure it would be there for me. Now, when I have it, I'm fearful about how long we will be together. Sometimes I go through periods of feeling more secure and grounded, more self-contained. In those times, I appreciate it and what it gives to me. Other times, I obsessively grasp for it, then feel guilty and shameful about my desperation. I punish myself for my greedy behavior.*
>
> *I'm also afraid of the consequences of having too much of it. I'd say we're always in a battle for control.*
>
> *My financial stress also gets between us. I have a dream I can make enough money someday that I can just put the price tag aside and enjoy our time together.*

Today it's sounds something like this:

> *We generally have a very respectful and symbiotic relationship. It nourishes me, and I honor it. We see each other at fairly regular times throughout the day, and while sometimes I dream up amazing things we can do together,*

most of the time I enjoy our pretty calm day-to-day relationship.

I don't think about it as much as I used to, yet I feel a deep bond with it. Sometimes I get a little bored and feel like I need to spice it up a bit – you know, add some variety. But I enjoy learning new things about it and have really come to understand how misunderstood it is. I feel like we've really come to understand and enjoy one another.

It's fun to look back and see the growth of our relationship! We've been through a lot together!

So much for my metaphorical growth. Let's take a journey to explore this odd, beautiful, and complex kinship we have with our primary relationship, food.

INTRODUCTION

I remember the drive well. I looked ahead to the horizon and told my dear friend, Holly, that I was on a mission to heal my *gut.* I told her when I did, I would write a book about how I did it, so I could help others through their own transformation.

After being by my side during the most physically painful and emotionally distraught period of my life, she nodded with encouragement, "Do it, Mad," she said. "I believe in you."

I did not know this pursuit would lead me down a path that would radically redefine my relationship to my body, heart, and career. It became a pilgrimage that led me to different cultures around the world. It led me on a spiritual journey deep into the hidden side of the food industry as well as hidden truths of myself.

At the time, I did not know how deeply seated the damaging belief systems around food were inside of me, in my community, and in the world at large. I did not know I would undertake a mission that contends with the largest, richest, and most powerful entities on Earth, as well as some of the deepest, darkest fears and insecurities housed within myself and countless others.

I did not realize what a charged topic food really is, nor how it carries lessons of courage, culture, racism, sexism, spirituality, and sexuality. That it holds the keys to some of the most pressing existential threats of our time, as we face both a public health crisis and eminent environmental collapse. Both of which are directly linked to our habits and beliefs about what we consume.

I've spent the last fifteen years studying food from a multitude of perspectives including nutrition, agriculture, culinary traditions, traditional cultures, food economics, health education, and mind-body practices. The first few years were spent motivated largely by my own healing process. The latter I spent applying what I had learned along the way to help others on a similar journey to transform their health and life.

I have run on the hamster wheel of seemingly endless pharmaceutical medications, as well as exploring many alternative and complementary health practices. Along the way I discovered and fell in love with Ayurveda, a system of health stemming from ancient India. Ayurveda, and its sister science, yoga, radically transformed my health. I became, and continue to be, a clinical practitioner of Ayurveda. Its wisdom is infused throughout this book, for which I take no credit. I am simply a vehicle for sharing it.

I now understand there are countless systems of medicine in existence today, each with expansive benefits as well as inherent limitations. I take pieces from every tradition I interact with, and I enjoy and understand their interconnectedness and contextual relevance.

It's clear to me that food is part of a much bigger picture than the common narratives around it such as calories, taste, and nutrition. It reaches into the most primal parts of our being and touches our highest aspirations as humans. It takes on unnecessary meanings and belief systems and has been used as an antagonizing force in both personal and collective ways. It also has the potential to offer copious benefits to the health and happiness of our bodies, minds, communities, and planet.

This book is written for you if you would like to change your *relationship* with food. It is not a dietary theory. My intention is to offer you a breath of fresh air as you explore this vast and dynamic topic within yourself.

I share candidly about my own journey through grueling chronic digestive issues paired with a persistent eating disorder, as well as stories of others I have worked with.

I also share the pivotal experiences and knowledge that remodeled and reinspired my life with food.

In an effort to illustrate both wide-angle and microcosmic perspectives, I highlight both scientific and esoteric wisdom. I offer questions of reflection to invite you to confront taboo topics, unveil hidden connections in your life's history, and activate a passionate and embodied sense of self. Through this exploration, you can consciously create a new, deeply satisfying relationship with food.

~

Our relationship with food is complicated. People have many different and sometimes contrasting experiences. I do not expect to capture all of them in this book, but I attempt to address many of them.

You will likely find that some experiences, feelings, and realizations resonate with you as you read, while some will not. I encourage you to notice the ones that do, those lightbulb moments, small or large, and explore them. Ponder the questions posed as writing prompts or share and explore with a friend or partner.

Talk out loud or audio-record yourself as you speak. Simply sit with them in meditation.

Just like a romantic partner is a reflection of you, so is your relationship with food. It reflects your connection to receive sustenance, engage pleasure, and unapologetically offer your authentic self to the world.

PART I

SUSTENANCE

I will never forget the short but powerful pause, then his deep, calm voice said to me, "Madison, food is good."

There was another pause between us. I took a deep breath. His words resonated, like the season's first echo of thunder. Right then and there, I became aware of the deep-seated belief I had hardwired into my mind that food was in some way "bad."

Childhood thoughts flash in front of me – the ballerina's diet of chicken broth and cocaine, my mother's challenge with her weight, my family's history of obesity, my embarrassment at the checkout counter growing up on food stamps. My mind was flooded with messages nurtured and encouraged through TV, movies, and magazines about how I should look, how much I should think about my weight, and how food surely makes me fat unless I learn to restrict myself.

Through the pain I hear the words "food is good." Saying those words to myself, I viscerally feel a weight lifted from me. My body begins to calm, to become grounded and lighter. The tension in my jaw relaxes as does the tightness in my stomach.

"You're right," I say as I laugh at the truth, "Food *is* good."

And this is my last bulimic episode. Ever!

For years I failed. For years I had punished myself. For years I repeated the same resolution, "I'll never do it again."

Over time I became more open about my experience with food. As I did, I noticed how many people were suffering from some sort of disordered eating. While bulimia may seem extreme to you, I have come to realize it's just a dot on the spectrum of disordered eating on which a tremendous number of people comprise a very diverse range of expressions.

The vast majority of my female friends and clients have experienced some deep-seated challenge with food throughout their life. Men struggle as well, though it's less talked about. This includes my father, who had a heart attack and a quintuple bypass when he was only thirty-nine years old. He radically changed his diet after recognizing the direct effect his food choices had on the health of his heart and the length of his life. He grew up in the Midwest of the United States, where "city chicken" – breaded and fried pork chops on a stick – remains a family favorite. After a near-death experience, he veered away from many cultural and familial "norms" he adopted in his youth.

I felt very alone and self-critical in my distraught eating history, but I have come to understand that we truly have a culture-wide "eating disorder" that can be seen from many angles. For example, eating habits are intensely personal and express our deepest feelings of longing, desire, fear, and comfort. They are tied intimately to feelings and habits we observe in our parents and family members. [1]

These habits are also collective, expressing the social, economic, and racial disparities that fuel the growth and distribution of food worldwide. Food is personal and political and everything in between.

In fact, we live in a world with rampant food inequality. It was reported in 2017 that one in four people globally were considered moderately or severely food insecure. That is 1.9 billion people. Of that, 22 percent of children were considered stunted, which is an indicator of severe malnutrition and considered irreversible after the first thousand days of a child's life.

1 Porges, Stephen W, and Deb Dana, *Clinical Applications of the Polyvagal Theory: The Emergence of Polyvagal-Informed Therapies (Norton Series on Interpersonal Neurobiology)* (New York: WW Norton & Company, 2018).

This can have irreversible cognitive and physical impacts throughout their life.[2]

In the developed world, food is more plentiful, leading to diseases of excess. Poor-quality, industrialized, packaged and prepared food is filled with empty calories and loaded with additives, chemicals, and antibiotics. These off-the-shelf, processed foods have become the accepted and normal diet for most households.

In 2019, over 20 percent of adults in each of the 50 U.S. states self-reported as obese. This can be attributed to the increasingly sedentary lifestyle of the average American but is mostly from unhealthy food habits.[3]

Heart disease and cancer continue to top the charts as leading causes of death in the U.S., and diabetes is steadily on the rise. Heart disease and diabetes are considered preventable by diet and lifestyle, and many cancers have been shown to be related to poor dietary choices or preventable by good ones.[4]

A few years ago, I accompanied a dear friend of mine to an appointment at the Children's Hospital in Los Angeles. As we found our way through the very opulently designed hospital, on our way from the lobby to the rheumatology department, I was astounded and disturbed to walk past a McDonald's – right there in the middle of the *Children's Hospital*!

We are poisoning our food supply, and our food supply is poisoning us. We often see that the same people who profit from our

2 Roser, Max. and Hannah Ritchie, "Hunger and Undernourishment," accessed May 25, 2021, https://ourworldindata.org/hunger-and-undernourishment#too-little-height-for-age-stunting

3 Centers for Disease Control and Prevention, "Adult Obesity Prevalence Maps," accessed June 29, 2021. https://www.cdc.gov/obesity/data/prevalence-maps.html

4 Amalia Waxman,"WHO Global Strategy on Diet, Physical Activity and Health," *Food and Nutrition Bulletin* 25, no.(3 (January 2004):), 292-302.

eating habits are the ones creating the standards. We have a problem here.

I live in a country where there are stretches hundreds of miles long that are considered "food deserts," where fresh produce cannot be found. It's clear that both our supply chain and our demand chain of food are loaded with imbalances.

For a lot of people, eating is a chore. For others, it's a guilty pleasure, and for many, a luxury. We project all sorts of other meanings onto food. We use it to reward and punish ourselves and our children. We stress eat and stress "don't eat".

It's no wonder, for so many of us, food has become something that is *not good.*

Yet, food is something that is supposed to nourish us physically, mentally, and spiritually. It feeds all our senses. It sustains us in a natural cycle that is inherently symbiotic.

Food is deeply tied to cultural and ancestral roots. As a woman, my food habits will directly impact my grandchildren through my DNA and its epigenetic expression. Each female child is born with about two million eggs already in her ovaries, grown with the DNA and nourishment she received in utero. This means the diet of a pregnant woman not only affects the developing child, it also affects the seeds of that child's future children. In essence, we are made up of not only what we eat but also what our grandmothers ate![5]

What once, only a few generations ago, came straight from the garden to our plates, now comes wrapped in about three layers of safety plastic, usually shipped from hundreds or thousands of miles away. That

---

5 Christopher Wanjek, "Your Diet Affects Your Grandchildren's DNA, Scientists Say," accessed January 29, 2021, https://www.livescience.com/21902-diet-epigenetics-grandchildren.html

plastic then ends up in the ocean which then poisons or kills our marine life, an important source of our food supply and an ecosystem we are all dependent on whether we consume aquatic animals or not.[6]

While there is rhyme and reason for this—safety, economics, efficiency, lawsuits, convenience – it's clear we've created a complex web and an eroding landscape.

If you find yourself challenged in your relationship with food, don't overlook the sensitivity you may have to the absurdity of our societal relationship to it. It's clear we've created a complex web and an eroding landscape that threatens the well-being of the Earth. If you find yourself challenged or feel anxiety in your relationship with food, examine your role as a consumer pressured by industry and culture to succumb to these absurdities that have evolved in the food industry over the last 100 years.

~

Food in its most primal essence is sustenance. It's given first through your mother's placenta, then through your mother's milk, and then through the gifts of Mother Earth through plants and animals.

Each primal role of food has both constructive and destructive sides of it, depending on how we relate to it. The *light* refers to engaging food as sustenance in a balanced way. The *shadow* emerges from our unconscious desires of attachment and aversion, leading to imbalance.

6 Gianna Andrews, "Plastics in The Ocean affecting Human Health," accessed September 29, 2021, https://serc.carleton.edu/NAGTWorkshops/health/case_studies/plastics.html

The light:

A well-nourished body is a foundation for good health. It encourages proper growth and healthy aging. It is comforting and nurturing. Its abundance is forthcoming, and with gratitude, we take what we need to sustain us. We encourage healthy systems inside of our body, and in the world outside of ourselves.

The shadow:

When too much sustenance is consumed, either out of fear or out of greed, our bodies and mind become a garden for disease to flourish. When we take more than what we need, our system is overwhelmed, and our channels are blocked. We perpetuate unsustainable systems that feed *dis-ease* in ourselves and others.

When sustenance is rejected or unavailable, we become depleted. The body's systems become fragile and start to break down. As we neglect ourselves, we are not able to fully show up for others in our lives.

What is your relationship to food as sustenance? How do you experience the light and/or shadow side of it? Note: You may, or likely, experience both.

Restorative Food Practices

My business partner and I had a very well-thought-out "food list" we would often give clients at our Ayurvedic Health Clinic. Ayurveda (pronounced eye-yur-**vay**-duh) is a system of health that stems from traditional East Indian medicine. It is thought to be the longest continuously practiced system of health in the world.[7]

7 Perel, Esther, *Mating in Captivity: Reconciling the Erotic and the Domestic* (New York: HarperCollins, 2006).

Ayurveda utilizes very sophisticated herbal remedies, and also emphasizes the role diet and lifestyle play in both preventing and healing disease.

Our food list was very straightforward and told our clients, from an Ayurvedic perspective, what foods we recommended they eat, shouldn't eat, or should eat in moderation. The sheet was personalized for each client with some common themes and was designed to help heal whichever ailments the client came in to address. While some people had great results with it, many did not.

Oftentimes people who would not identify as having "disordered eating" would express a trauma response to the food list. They'd do really well for a period of time, then drop off their regimen – often around the holidays, or while traveling. Their new habits would collapse. They would indulge in their previous habits and then feel guilt, shame, fear, anger– a whole slew of different emotions pointed both inward at themselves and outward at us!

Sometimes it would lead a person to recognize their emotional triggers around withholding desires. I often heard, "Whoa, that was intense. I had no idea how powerful my feelings of *deprivation* were!" Or "how addicted I am to…."

Sometimes it would make them realize how much better they felt on the diet than they did when they fell off. With this recognition, they would often reengage their healing regimen and have great success. In the second round, they typically preferred the diet because they *felt* better, not because it was something they had been "told" to do.

For some, the experience of receiving such a detailed directive for dietary change was simply overwhelming. There was too much change and their old habits were too ingrained to transform overnight. It intimidated them, and the fear of failing made them feel hopeless.

For others, the mere concept of a "diet" was frightening and triggered very real and intense feelings and memories associated with disordered eating, challenges with body image, or food scarcity.

Observing my clients' responses to our early attempts to change their dietary habits, I learned that these patterns are much more complex than simply following directives.

I have come to realize there is a part of each of our psyches that wants the quick formula for success in whatever realm we're feeling stuck or unsatisfied. I often tell people who come in to see me for chronic health conditions that, while it's an inconvenient truth, there really is no such thing as a "magic pill" – even a natural one.

The modern world has reinforced the notion that there is some technological invention or medication that can fix any problem, any ailment, any time. As a patient, I want to be given the magic pill, and as a health practitioner, I want to be able to offer it! However, we are continually disappointed when we are reminded over and over again that our problems persist.

There are always two ways to approach health and disease – either directly, with brute force, or by seeking to restore balance. Both ways are valid. Both have their strengths and limitations. Our allopathic (modern) medical system typically takes the first approach. Ayurveda, and other holistic modalities, emphasize the importance of the second.

For example, when you have a fast-growing cancer in the body, any form of medicine needs to be extremely powerful, penetrating, and fast-moving. This is also applicable when you're facing a threat like a house fire. To survive, either by getting out of the house or by putting the fire out, the action needs to be extremely powerful and quick. In these cases, harsh substances or actions, such as chemotherapy or fire-retardants, will often save the day. They also generally have consequences or side-effects that need to be dealt with later, but the success of surviving the intense threat can be worth the restoration efforts.

You don't need these same extreme countermeasures for every situation. The same way you don't need to grab the fire extinguisher when the doorbell rings unexpectedly, you wouldn't use chemotherapy drugs to treat an acne condition. There are better options for addressing the potential threat – installing an alarm system, or by purifying the body through a lighter and cleaner diet to clear congestion in the skin. Once in a while, calling on the warrior to do battle is necessary. Most of the time, it's not.

Similar to our modern approach to human health, we see an analogous pattern in our industrial food production. World over, we are seeing disturbing trends in the depletion of agricultural soil that has been farmed through monoculture farming (planting one crop year-after-year on the same plot) and pesticide use. These practices, while productive in the short run, lead to nutrient-depleted soil that degrades the yield of crops, the nutrient density of food, and our regional and global ecosystems. This is an example of taking the brute force approach to our food production.

Similar to how restorative health seeks to restore balance to the individual, restorative agriculture seeks to restore balance to the ecosystem. Regenerative farming practices prioritize the health of the soil. They diversify crops. They build systems that use both food and waste products from plants and animals symbiotically. This approach, while admittedly more complex and harder to scale quickly, creates a more sustainable, vibrant, and nutritious environment for food to be grown.

Just like the comprehensive approach required to restore balance to an entire ecosystem, most chronic health conditions require us to honor the relationship between interdependent systems body. Restoring health typically requires a change across a mu of habits including diet, exercise, biorhythms, stress and even h relate to others.

Restoring our health in this manner generally takes longer, requires more participation from us, but has more sustainable results and less side-effects – sometimes none at all.

Brute force generates quick results and has appropriate uses. If overused or misused, however, it creates damage and destruction. Even when we use it appropriately, after the battle is won, we have to rebuild our systems in a new, healthier way. This is commonly overlooked.

My Story of Eating

In the spirit of vulnerability and turning messes into messages, I've overcome some pretty big ones (messes) in my life.

I remember being intensely ashamed during my episodes of bulimia. It always started with a secret anxiety – a fearful decoction of failing, getting fat, being broke, and being alone. It drove me to scavenge for food, escalating in intensity, towards anything I could get my hands on that was sweet, fatty, carb-heavy goodness.

What I consumed didn't even need to taste good. I would binge eat Doritos and Reese's peanut butter cups when I babysat. I would steal fancy chocolates from my roommates' pantry and refrigerator. I would go to the gas station and buy sour cream donuts and potato chips, and stuff my face with it.

I would keep going and going until I couldn't ingest anymore, and then I would make myself throw it all back up.

The first time, it wasn't that bad, but after a few rounds of this, a few days in a row, I felt like total garbage. At first, I told myself it was just once. Then just a phase. It wasn't until years had gone by with these periodic episodes that I came to recognize my habits as an eating disorder. Years afterward I came to understand and feel compassion for the traumas that led to the belief systems I carried and to the self-deprecating actions that came from them.

My poor relationship with food didn't start then. It started back when I was a toddler. One day, I played in a grassy field that was recently sprayed with pesticides. The experience left me ill. I was treated with large doses of antibiotics and steroids. This in turn affected my immune system and my gut health, which at the time, was neither medically understood, nor publicly discussed.

Afterwards, as the story goes, I would just refuse to eat. My mother would manually open my mouth, and my father would stuff the food in for me.

Understandably, I didn't feel well.

I did not know how to communicate my discomfort, other than by refusing food. So, I tried to use the universal language of boundaries – yes or no.

My parents thought they were caring for me. Instead, I internalized my first experience of non-consent – how I chose what went in my body and what stayed outside.

That seemed to jump start a series of both physical repulsion to food and emotional control games around it. Later in life, those patterns of non-consent showed up in the way of "unwanted" sexual experiences, and emotionally violent relationship dynamics. Boundaries remained a challenging mystery to me, and food became a playground to explore and express my internal battle with them.

As an older child, I found all sorts of creative ways to avoid eating my vegetables and other things I didn't like. I was a notoriously picky eater. I'd bury food in napkins, put them in my pocket, then flush them down the toilet. I'd stuff my mouth with my dinner, then go to the bathroom and spit it out. I'd pretend to fall asleep at the TV dinner table. My dad would finally give up and take the food away, and my scheme would work. This is an example of the shadow side of sustenance – aversion to food.

My parents separated when I was four years old. My home with my mother was volatile and wrought with unhealthy dynamics. I understand now that food was one of my only bargaining tools in our power struggle. It was something I had some control over, in an atmosphere that felt totally out of control and often unsafe. I ran away from home when I was 16 and ended up living with my father for the remaining years of high school.

Fast-forward to age 20. I was sick again. I was reluctantly taking a growing cocktail of pharmaceutical medications. Each one seemed to lead to a side effect that led to another pill. My medley of seemingly unrelated health issues remained a mystery to every doctor I visited and a source of pain and confusion to me and my family.

I felt like an elderly person walking down the halls of my college dorm dressed in the body of a 20-year-old. I was suffering from severe digestive problems, chronic pain in my joints, and neurological pain down my arms and hands. I had heartburn, high cholesterol, asthma, and insomnia.

I genuinely felt like I was dying, degenerating. When people would ask me about my future career plans or if I wanted to be a mother, I remember answering that I didn't know if I would make it to thirty.

As my daily pill count added up, I was getting worse and more hopeless. I hit a breaking point with the medical hamster wheel I had been spinning on since I was a child. I realized that *I* was the common denominator in all of it, and I would need to change my life.

I was still a picky eater, but when my sister suggested I take gluten out of my diet, in an act of desperation, I did.

I started to learn about how food could be affecting my body and the chronic health conditions that ailed it. I had immediate results. My pain and inflammation lowered almost instantaneously. It stunned and inspired me. It set me on a journey to learn about food – its roots, its reality, and its healing potential.

A new door opened in front of my eyes. Behind it, I discovered foods I had never even heard of. The produce section of my local grocery store became a cornucopia of colorful delights that had been there all along.

As I started to learn about nutrition, read labels, and research where food came from, I was amazed by what was really in the food I was accustomed to eating – the chemicals, the preservatives, the sugar, the fillers. At the time, before the gluten-free craze began, gluten was in almost everything. It was in cranberry juice for God's sake! I was flabbergasted and curious – why?

Studying this strange phenomenon led me down a path of learning about the roots of, and agendas behind, food production. I started to learn about agricultural processes, and the economic and political forces at play behind the products we so casually pick off the shelf. I found myself spending hours per week at all types of grocery stores, reading labels, educating myself about food, and studying trends.

Learning about food sparked my curiosity of its agricultural roots. The summer after my junior year of college, I got a job as one of three interns running the organic farm at The Colorado College. This luscious plot of land in the backyard of the president's house was home to a robust vegetable garden, a chicken coop, a beehive, and a newly planted orchard with a variety of young fruit trees.

I was a total novice. I knew nothing about farming except for the idealistic understanding of its importance I had learned from reading and watching documentaries as part of my independent food investigation.

The farm was run solely by me, two other women, a handful of occasional volunteers, and overseen by our faculty sponsor. By the end of the summer, it was an edible paradise that offered food to our CSA (community supported agriculture), our college cafeteria, and local farmers markets. It also offered a destination for young children and a group of "at-risk" teenagers to come learn about farming and get their hands and bodies into the craft.

It was truly a life changing experience for me.

It was the closest I had ever lived to nature. It amazed me how much food three people could generate on a small plot of land, and how much hard work it took to do so.

It taught me lessons about the interdependence of natural life through agricultural practices like *permaculture* and *companion planting*. These practices show us how, when we honor symbiotic relationships, species work together to help each other survive and thrive. A "three sisters" garden is a classic example. For centuries, corn, beans, and squash have been cornerstones of Native American agriculture and culinary traditions. They are known as *the three sisters*. These crops complement each other both in the garden and on the plate; they are traditionally grown together, eaten together, and celebrated together.

Corn's tall stature acts as a trellis for the beans to climb up, so they do not have to compete on the garden floor with sprawling squash vines. Beans, in turn, provide nitrogen to fertilize the soil while also stabilizing the tall corn during very heavy winds. Beans are nitrogen-fixers, meaning they host rhizobia on their roots which take nitrogen, a vital nutrient for plants, from the air and convert it to be absorbable by plant roots. Squash finishes out the support circle by providing large leaves that shade the ground for all three plants, which helps retain soil moisture and prevent weeds.

These three plants, which have qualities that could destroy each other as they compete for resources, work together to create a thriving environment for growth when they are planted and cared for together. This contrasts the typical modern mono-cropping farming method where one crop at a time is planted in vast plots of land.

Learning about and experiencing the companionship of the three sisters made me recognize how I longed for companionship and sisterhood in the same way. It made me reflect on how we can achieve more when we put our hearts and heads together, than when we just add the sum of our parts or compete for the spotlight. Cultural diversity, when honored, creates thriving communities.

How ironic that I ended up with my bare feet in this outdoor paradise with two other beautiful women, from completely different backgrounds, with unique skills and desires. Our skin was different, our ancestries were different, we were different shapes and sizes, and we had never spoken before, yet we shared a bond we didn't even know we had. We, too, were *three sisters*.

While working on the farm, I remembered what it felt like to play outside. I faced many of my first-world fears of bugs and critters and of simply being dirty. I developed a sensory relationship with where food came from – the smells, the colors, the textures. I learned about new edible plants, and suddenly I liked foods that I had always turned away.

I learned about the history of foods and seeds, and the people who sowed them. I learned of the mass carnage of the plants, animals, people, and land that has, and continues to be, colonized, sabotaged, and overtaken for material pursuits. I came to understand how deeply tied we are, without even realizing it, to the trauma that our land and our ancestors have both experienced and perpetrated.

While working on the farm, I also fell in love with the beauty of wildness. I witnessed fugitive plants – ones that were never planted – sprout up in the walkways and perimeters of the garden. Their seeds were just waiting for the right environment in which to come to life. They showed me even when cultivated, nature cannot be controlled. Those seeds that were planted long ago can sprout when you least expect them to – in the garden, and in ourselves.

I gained a respect for the whole process from seed to seed that contains so much wisdom of life itself.

Food really began to take on new meanings for me. While I was not free of all of my emotional triggers, I noticed that food was holding a much softer, less threatening, and more nurturing quality than it ever had before. As I nurtured the sustenance of the garden, I too accepted and created sustenance that fed me – body, mind, and soul.

I continue to seek experiences like this, experiences that connect me to nature and to myself. I also continue to wade through ideas and constructs that build the worldview that informs my reality.

~

I hid my eating disorder for many years. In college, I ventured to tell a couple of my close friends about it on two separate occasions. I was surprised by their reactions. There really weren't any.

At the time, I felt confused, uncertain why my friends were so unconcerned with what I was going through. Looking back, I understand their apathetic response likely had nothing to do with me but was expressive of their own challenging relationships with food. I often hear similar stories from my clients.

I was surprised when, a few years later, a friend I had confided in invited me into an open conversation about my disordered eating. How refreshing!

It's interesting to look back at these conversations and observe who engaged honestly with me and who did not. I found plenty of friends who encouraged the disordered relationship. This was largely unconscious, simply because they had their own form of it.

Imagine a woman who experiences a traumatic event in her life and begins to lose weight. Her friends, noticing her trim figure, shower her with compliments. What a confusing experience – to be, on the one hand, praised for attaining an idealized physique and, on the other hand, suffer the symptoms of extreme psychological pain of a dysfunctional eating disorder. Unfortunately, it is rare to have a conscious conversation about the dysfunctional patterns most people are experiencing.

It is easy to participate in the normalized rhetoric around food and dieting. I hid the "darker" side of my eating disorder, thinking I was more or less alone in my indulgent suffering.

Once I began to talk about it openly, I realized hiding actually fueled my behavior. Later in life, as I explored my erotic desires, I discovered "forbidden" things are at the top of the list – more about that later. Over the years I've found when I honestly share my experiences, many people suddenly feel safe enough to talk about theirs. Contrary to my fears of vulnerability, my hidden shame and dysfunction with food was not unique to me.

~

I knew I had landed somewhere special when, after a recent move to Los Angeles, I found myself sitting in the home of a learned yogi. He knows not just of the postures of yoga, but also of the healing powers of a disciplined mind and the callings of the soul.

He looked at me deeply, and with a coarse, compassionate voice asked, "So, what's your story?" As I answered, he listened to much more than my words. He reached over, gave me a cookie, and commanded, "Here, eat!"

I immediately started down my beloved list of questions and explanations about food that I had been refining for years in order to preserve my temperamental gut and newfound nutritional competence.

"Thanks," I said, "But what's it made of? I'm allergic to gluten so I can't have..." and then caught my thoughts and paused.

I decided to eat the cookie anyway. While I was supposed to be allergic to this capacious mound of sweet vegan spelt chocolate chip goodness, I wasn't. I experienced no adverse reaction at all – no stomach ache, no headache, no joint pain.

That day, it was clear to me there was much more to this picture than *gluten* as the culprit of my digestive problems.

I kept coming back, knocking on his door, expecting to do "yoga." Instead, I was fed. We did some of what most people would consider yoga, a series of postures on a mat, but for the next year, we spent most of our time talking and eating. I cried my life out as we sat on his crimson couch, eating cookies, pie, vegan sushi rolls, and all sorts of other heavenly foods. I radically changed my lifestyle and began to unwind patterns of *dis-ease* in both my body and mind.

It was clear to me that I was looking not only to heal but for meaning and purpose. Intuitively, I knew there was much more to life than what meets the blind eye, and that my health problems expressed something much deeper than the physical symptoms I was experiencing.

I came to understand that yoga is not just postures on a mat, but rather a practice of consciousness that extends to every facet of life. This includes what you eat and how you eat it. I began a journey that would transform my life and that has transformed many others.

In the coming years, I learned how to use food as medicine. I learned how to understand the qualities of food. I learned how to use and understand the six tastes and their relevance to health and cooking. I learned how different types of heating and cooking changed the qualities of food, and the importance of not just what you eat, but how well you digest it. I learned about a whole world of medicinal herbs and spices. I truly fell in love with food and cooking.

A decade later, food is still a centerpiece of my life – in the programs I design for my clients, in the conversations I have as an environmental activist, and in the meals that I prepare for friends and clients. People describe me as having "magic hands" that not only seem to know how to heal through touch, but how to heal through food.

My past is riddled with disordered eating, yet the world of food has gone from one of my greatest challenges to one of my most valued assets.

Your Story of Eating

Recognizing where, when, and how your current relationship with food manifested is an important step. It can help you identify your habitual eating patterns and develop self-compassion for food-related behavioral oddities in your life. Knowing the root of your relationship with food can stimulate you to question your eating habits in ways you might not have ever thought of.

You may notice some themes in my story that you relate to. You may recognize how the roots of your eating habits trace back to your upbringing – your parents' habits, the media, the culture you grew up in, financial stability, activities you participated in, or big events that shaped you.

From a neuroscientific perspective, the first thing that reaches our consciousness proves to have the most powerful effect.[8] For example, our initial impression of a situation or event we hear about on the news immediately becomes our baseline belief about it.[9] Every other subsequent perspective is compared suspiciously to that baseline belief. We can understand how dramatic political schisms can be fueled by media and propaganda. We can also see how our habits and beliefs can be absorbed from our early caretakers. No matter how many other perspectives we get as we age, the voice of our parents seems to be logged subconsciously as our baseline worldview no matter how hard we try to eliminate it.[10]

8 Boris, Kotchoubey, "Human Consciousness: Where Is It From and What Is It For," *Frontiers in Psychology*, no. 9 (April, 2018): 567.

9 Camila Domonoske, "Students Have 'Dismaying' Inability to Tell Fake News from Real, Study Finds," accessed May 31, 2021, https://www.npr.org/sections/thetwo-way/2016/11/23/503129818/study-finds-students-have-dismaying-inability-to-tell-fake-news-from-real

10 Boris Kotchoubey, "Human Consciousness: Where Is It From and What Is It For," *Frontiers in Psychology* 9 (April, 2018): 567.

In a survey I conducted, 45 percent responded that one or both of their parents had some form of disordered eating. Interestingly 23 percent responded "I don't know." One respondent shared with me that the question made her wonder why and how she did not know.

She asked, "Why was it never talked about? Or never thought about? What was pushed under the rug and hidden away?"

What concepts and behaviors around food did you take from your father? How about your mother?

Which of these things would you like to hold on to? Which would you like to let go of?

If recognition of these roots brings up feelings of anger, resentment, or anxiety, I encourage you to notice them.

I don't want to create a blame-fest here – in fact, quite the opposite. By connecting the dots of your story of eating, you can bring clarity to how your relationship with food has influenced your life and visa versa. As an adult, you can take full responsibility for the way you have responded to these events in your life.

As you unravel your history of eating, you have two choices: (1) you can remain a victim of the past, or (2) you can develop self-compassion for the way you responded to the circumstances at hand. The ability to take full responsibility for your story gives you the power to accept the present. This is the only way to change your future.

Let's take an example. My mother often didn't make enough money to buy us food. For periods of time, we survived on food stamps or donations from community organizations. I can either choose to feel victimized by being a child of a financially irresponsible mother and blame her for that piece of my disordered eating. Or I can recognize that I responded to the situation by embodying a feeling of food-scarcity.

This is a completely understandable response. I can feel a deep sense of compassion for the small girl who felt hunger and fear because vital resources were limited. I can also see how I took that feeling into my early adulthood, a feeling which informed the choices I made about food.

My experience with scarcity fueled my binge-eating episodes. When I had an abundance of food available to me, like at other people's houses, I often anxiously ate more than I needed. Whether real or imagined, I unconsciously feared I might not have enough later.

By taking responsibility for my response, I have the opportunity to make a different choice the next time I am presented with a similar feeling or circumstance.

The word *responsibility* is the union of *response* and *ability.* Taken together, responsibility means that we have the ability to choose our response for that which we take responsibility for. Radical honesty mixed with self-responsibility is a powerful combination when it comes to healing. Add *self-compassion* to this mix and you have a true healing cocktail!

So, what is *your* story of eating?

As you recall, whether you're reflecting silently, out loud, or in writing, I encourage you to *get real.* Get explicit. What are the dirty details of your eating life? What are the roots? The major players? The real feelings that correspond with your experience. Get it out, somehow, either in writing or verbally. If you write it, perhaps share it with someone in your life with whom you feel safe.

As you do this, notice if you use passive language such as "this happened to me so now I am like this…" When these types of phrases surface, reframe them into sentences like "I experienced ____, and I responded to that by ___."

For example:

My parents fought incessantly at the dinner table, which gave me a negative association to eating around other people.

Rephrase as:

I experienced deep feelings of anxiety and loneliness at the dinner table when my parents fought. I responded by resisting family meals and preferred eating food outside the house. Now I often create ways to enjoy my favorite foods by myself, sometimes even in secret. I have not created a family culture of eating together.

I encourage you to keep your exploration honest and light-hearted. I don't mean for you to ignore heavy experiences or emotions. I don't mean just "think positive." I mean maintain an air of self-compassion and playfulness. This topic can be challenging, wrought with both positive and negative associations. Remind yourself that it's complex. There is no right or wrong here.

Each part of your story is ultimately here to help you learn and become a more authentic you. Laugh at yourself. Bring light to a dark shadow. Start to enjoy the odd but amazing pleasure of being a hungry human.

You might explore:

What do you consider your main avenues of sustenance (money, love, food, status, attention…)?

What habits or beliefs have you experienced in relationship to each of your parents around nourishment?

What are your cultural narratives and ancestral links to primal sustenance?

You are What You ~~Eat~~ Digest

I remember the days of making my "superfood" smoothie, loaded with at least ten of the most nutrient-dense foods I had gleaned from the internet and a stack of nutrition books. I mixed the ingredients with eager anticipation of their *super* health benefits – you know, anti-inflammatory, loaded with omegas, vitamins, minerals, and antioxidants. It would look something like a cold, thick, brownish-green sludge of almond milk, yogurt, chia seeds, flax seeds, spirulina, almond butter, goji berry, raw cacao, banana, kale, pea protein powder, ice and healthfully sweetened, of course, with dates and agave nectar.

It tasted about as good as it looked, but my belief in how *healthy* it was overpowered the aftertaste of creamy, chewy dirt.

Little did I realize that my *superfood* smoothie was actually *super-too-hard* for my body to digest. I was likely absorbing very little of the nutrients that I'd loaded into my meal.

It was certainly a far reach from the cheese, bread, meat, and sugar that had comprised most of my diet for the previous twenty years. Fueled by innocent enthusiasm, desperation, and great marketing by food manufacturers, my early days as a novice nutrition junky were like a gateway drug. My quest for nutrition opened a door to a whole world of foods I didn't even know existed. This ultimately led me to a much deeper understanding of the role that food plays in the body and mind.

My health leapt forward when I learned nutrition is not just about *what* you eat, but *how well you digest* what you eat. I could eat a cornucopia of the most nutrient dense foods in the world, but I would not receive the benefits of their bounty if I could not digest them well.

Until recently, the mainstream medical community resisted the notion that the gut and the mind are connected, and that what we eat contributes directly to chronic diseases. Now, an abundance of research has emerged that intimately links the gut and mind, the immune system, and the inflammatory response. I see a reference to the gut microbiome and the brain-gut connection in popular media almost every day.

A healthy gut is a prerequisite to strong digestion. As a whole, our modern lifestyles, diet, stress and personal histories have compromised the functioning of our gut. Healing our digestion requires taking a holistic and integrative approach that seeks to restore balance to our whole system. This is a central pillar of Ayurveda.

Despite its roots in the Sanskrit language, which was foreign to me, Ayurveda felt like a language I had known for lifetimes. When I began my study, I felt at last connected to a truth that I knew but no one was talking about. Ayurveda is the study of the laws of nature, applied to human health, our planet and its inhabitants, all of which we depend upon for life and medicine.

Ayurveda is a living science meant to evolve as the cultural and biological landscape of our world evolves. Ayurveda does not treat disease, it treats people. It looks at each human being as a unique set of experiences, constitutions, and patterns of balance. It assesses qualities of strength, resilience, and inherent spirituality irrespective of religion. It uses remedies found in nature, in physical form, in rhythm, and in energetics, to help guide us to a point of balance.

Physical remedies: food, herbs, minerals, exercise
Rhythm: biorhythms, daily routines, seasonal routines
Energetics: elemental forces, metaphysics, clearing subtle channels

Learning and applying Ayurvedic principles of health helped me heal the deep-seated conditions I was suffering from, including my chronic pain and digestive imbalances.

"The goal of life is to make your heartbeat match the heartbeat of the universe, to match your nature with Nature."
– Joseph Campbell

Our bodies are made up of the transformed matter and energy of the food we eat. In Ayurveda, the word for diet is *Ahara*. Ahara means everything you intake – what you eat, drink, breathe, and perceive. This elevates the concept of diet far beyond just the calories you ingest. That means that the meal you ate today is part of your diet, but so is the Instagram feed you read while you ate it. The more intimately I study health, the body, and people's relationship with food, the more clearly this is reinforced.

This expanded definition of diet can be seen by how the systems of the body interrelate. The food you eat gets macerated by your gastrointestinal system. The liquid you drink gets assimilated by your renal, urinary, and lymph systems. The air you breathe, and anything mixed in with it – like pollution, smoke, or aromas – gets filtered through the respiratory system. Your mental observations get taken in by the nervous system.

While old medical models describe the body mechanically as systems that relate largely independently from one another, we now know these systems each communicate and co-exist with each other within a multidimensional system that make up the human body and mind. Each system – and the food that feeds it – impacts the overall functioning of the whole body. By looking at the ways the gut connects to the rest of the body, we can understand this magnificent interdependence.

For instance, the immune cells in your gut make up the largest part of your immune system. There are more immune cells that reside in the lining of your gut than there are in your blood or bone marrow.

The lining of your gut is loaded with endocrine cells that contain up to 20 different types of hormones. If you combined all these, it would be greater than all your other endocrine organs – your gonads, thyroid gland, pituitary gland, and the adrenal glands – combined!

The gut is also filled with gut microbiota – the bacteria, archaea, fungi, and viruses that live inside the gut. There are 100,000 times more of these microbes in your gut than there are people on Earth. They are the ecosystem responsible for what you crave, and to a large degree, how you digest what you eat.[11]

The gut is also the largest storage facility for serotonin in our body. Serotonin is a vital hormone that stabilizes mood and produces feelings of well-being and happiness. It enables cells in the brain and the nervous system to communicate with one another, and therefore has a systemic impact on the entire body. It affects our emotions, our sleep, and our appetite. Amazingly, 95 percent of the body's serotonin is stored in your gut![12] Serotonin is also the main target of the major class of antidepressants, the serotonin reuptake inhibitors. This is why diet, and the health of our gut, has such a significant impact on our state-of-mind. Similarly, our state-of-mind has a significant impact on our digestion.

11 Douglas. J. Davies, and Michael J. Thate, *Religion and the Individual: Belief, Practice, and Identity* (Basel: MDPI-Multidisciplinary Digital Publishing Institute, 2017).

12 Elder Mayer, *The Mind-Gut Connection: How The Hidden Conversation Within Our Bodies Impacts Our Mood, Our Choices, and Our Overall Health* (New York: Harper-Collins, 2018).

The function of our gut is perhaps the single most important facet to our trajectory of health or disease. Modern science is just now catching up to what Ayurveda, and many other traditional systems of medicine, have outlined for thousands of years.[13]

There is an appropriate time and place for all systems of medicine. Because of its integrative approach to health, Ayurveda is particularly effective when addressing chronic health conditions. According to the National Health Council, about 40 percent of the United States population suffers from chronic health conditions. Given our fast-paced lifestyles, relatively poor modern diet, and agitated state-of-mind, this statistic is no surprise.

Your body is literally made from the food you eat. But in order for food to become you, it must be *ingested*, *assimilated*, and *eliminated* properly. If there is an imbalance in any of these functions, even the best food won't become healthy tissue in your body.

So – what made my smoothie so hard to digest? It was too heavy, too cold, and made up of poor food combinations. In addition, my system was already compromised. My digestive fire, *agni*, was low. I didn't come to the table with a hot fire capable of burning up the raw, dense mud-shake I poured on top of it. What I couldn't digest sat in my digestive tract and became a toxin or passed through without being assimilated.

Transforming your relationship with your digestion is similar to that of training a puppy. It requires observation, discipline, consistency, and compassion. Your digestion, like the puppy, can become your adherent ally, or it can wreak havoc on virtually all aspects of your human experience.

---

13 Stephan C. Bischoff, "'Gut Health': A New Objective in Medicine?" *BMC Medicine* 9, no. 1 (March, 2011): 1-14.

Good digestion is the end result of an array of lifestyle habits, physical and mental. You are not just what you eat, you are what you digest. Eating good food, digesting it well, and enjoying it in a relaxed state are ingredients for a healthy diet.

The Four Pillars of Digestion: What, When, How, and How Much

Laura, an Iyengar yoga teacher and nutritionist in her early 30s, came to see me for a consultation. She described her diet as "blog-worthy" – she felt like she was doing everything right – and was perplexed as to why her severe digestive issues continued to worsen.

She was in severe pain every day. She constantly held her abdomen. Her bones and muscles ached, and she felt like going back to bed as soon as she woke up. She alternated between periods of constipation and diarrhea.

She ate lots of vegetables, mostly salads, and a good amount of organic free-range beef and fish. She was getting all the "nutrients" she thought she needed. She had been to countless medical practitioners who had suggested various medications and supplements. None of them worked. Some seemed to make it worse. Now she was trying to manage her pain and discomfort herself.

After I learned about her diet and life, I suspected that while she was eating nutrient dense foods, she was not digesting it. We put together a dietary protocol that I hoped would be easier for her system to *digest*, *assimilate*, and *eliminate* and would give her body the opportunity to heal.

The diet was simple. It consisted of things like *kitchari* – a delicious blend of rice, mung beans, vegetables, ghee, and spices, as well as soups, stews, and some nourishing sweet fruits. I asked her to avoid certain foods and eat others in abundance. I helped her regulate the timing of her meals and discard snacking. I recommended warm foods and drinks. I offered ayurvedic herbs and spices alongside her food to support her system. I prepared an herbal oil for her skin – the body's most absorbent organ – as a self-massage practice multiple times per week.

She carefully followed the protocol we drafted up. At first, it gave her some anxiety to eat different meals than her partner, but she soon realized her gut health was more important than his opinion of her diet. She noticed that their relationship improved as she felt better.

Within a couple of months, her stomach aches were completely gone. Her joint pain nearly subsided. She woke up with good energy and went back to teaching full-time. She continued to keep her diet simple and enjoyed both preparing and eating the food she made for herself.

Laura's story is a testament to how healthy eating is far more than just how many calories and nutrients we eat. We must also consider the quality, the timing, and the mindset in which we dine.

We break down eating into four basic categories:

***What*:** The physical quality of the food and its nutritional efficacy for you
***When*:** The timing, rhythm, and regularity of your meals
***How much*:** The quantity you take in
***How*:** The mindset and demeanor in which you eat

Each category is of *equal importance.*

Weight loss programs often focus solely on "how much," emphasizing caloric intake.

Modern nutrition adds the emphasis of "what." Specifically, the nutrient density, vitamin and mineral profile, and food categorization (carbohydrate, fat, protein, etc.).

Some diet trends, such as intermittent fasting, emphasize a fast between an early dinner and a late lunch the following day, focusing on "when."

The mindset, or "how," is definitely the neglected stepchild of nutritional guidance. It is one of the golden threads of this book.

Let's take a look at each one in a bit more detail.

***What:* The physical quality of the food and its nutritional efficacy for you**

Everything in nature is medicinal if used in the right way.
– Ayurvedic proverb

I have held onto a handful of these phrases that were gifted to me by teachers. They are like precious gems whose luminosity expands the deeper I look at them.

The properties of food are absolutely fascinating. If everything in nature is medicinal when used in the right way, then all food can either be a medicine, when used appropriately, or a toxin, when used inappropriately.

According to Ayurveda, each person is built with a unique constitution and with a digestive capacity that is made to support it. What is medicinal to one person can be poison to another.

People tend to categorize things as good or bad, healthy or unhealthy. However, any *real* food is neither all good nor all bad. Every "real" food item and ingredient has a nutritional profile, micro and macro, as well as qualities such as heating, cooling, acidic, alkaline, diuretic, and so on. Each food's unique combination makes up its flavor, its action on the body, and even its relationship to the environment in which it grows.[14]

It's pretty cool to recognize that there are foods that decrease blood pressure, and foods that increase it.

There are foods that cause diarrhea, and foods that stop it.

There are foods that cleanse the blood, and others that build it. There are foods that heal wounds, that reduce cholesterol, and reduce inflammation. There are foods that lower anxiety, and ones that help you sleep.

There are foods that help the body digest extra fat, others that help build bones. There are some that improve concentration, and others that act as aphrodisiacs!

The world of food is like a wild farm-acy of nature's medicine. It's spectacular if you really take this to heart! Every food you eat either helps or harms you.

In Ayurvedic medicine, foods and medicinal substances are based on five properties and include:

- Taste (*rasa*)
- Attributes (*guna*)
- Potency (*virya*)
- Post-digestive Affect (*vipaka*)
- Therapeutic Action (*karma*)

14 Eva. Glader, Matthew Fraser, Gerard Roemers, O. Sabag Muñoz, Erin Kennedy, and Peter Hirsch, "What are Macronutrients and Micronutrients," accessed April 20, 2021, https://www.getsmarter.com/blog/market-trends/what-are-macronutrients-and-micronutrients/

An elaborate study of these properties provides a comprehensive understanding of nutrition and is one of Ayurveda's great contributions to natural and holistic medicine.[15]

Studying and understanding the properties of food can be both magical and overwhelming. How are we supposed to know what is good for us and what isn't? There is no one-size-fits-all answer to this question. Differences in constitution, season, quality of food, stress level, digestive capacity, stage of life, time of day, and genetic factors can all impact which foods you need and how well you digest them.

Evaluating, in detail, the properties of individual foods and their effect on the unique individual is beyond the scope of this book, as my main goal here is to address our *relationship* with the food we eat. I will, however, outline general considerations in the coming sections. These are broken into two main sections: *Seeing Beyond Dietary Myths and Fads* and *Finding Foods That Nourish*. I have also included an *Ayurvedic Body Constitution Assessment* and corresponding food and lifestyle recommendations in the workbook section at the back of the book.

1. *Seeing Beyond Dietary Myths and Fads*

There have been many iterations of dietary trends in the western world. We've seen things like the low-fat diet, the Atkins diet, the Paleo diet, the keto diet, and the gluten-free diet. Each takes its turn in the spotlight of cultural relevance, endorsed by big-name celebrities, doctors, and motivational marketing. There is efficacy to them all when used in the right way. Taking gluten out of my diet for a period of time was an important part of healing my gut. The keto diet can be a very effective weight loss program for the right person. Some people benefit greatly from limiting grains in their diet.

15 Sanjay Pisharodi, *Acharya Vagbhata's Astanga Hrdayam: The Essence of Ayurveda (Vol. 1)* (South Carolina: CreateSpace Independent Publishing).

However, these dietary fads all tend to follow a similar trajectory. First, a study or dietary theory emerges. Then, it is used in a well-funded marketing campaign to allure the average person through their dualistic relationship to food.[9] Next, a whole industry of packaged products is created to cater to their grab-and-go food habits. Meanwhile, popular media broadcasts the message: "You are not good enough. Lose weight. Be more beautiful."

Generally, these "diets" make it all the way to the mainstream before warnings come out about the dangers, short-comings, or limited nature of their claims. They are quickly replaced by the next fad or co-exist in a cacophony of contradictory messages that keep many people in informational paralysis. "Fats are bad!" "Carbs are terrible!" "Meat is God!" "Meat is the devil!"

What's the truth? I guess I'll just eat whatever I want.

Meanwhile, a handful of industries profit from our debilitated relationship with food – generally, meat, dairy, sugar and packaged foods. And, of course, the packaging and transportation industries that support them. These industries are ideologically and financially linked to two of our country's biggest enterprises, large-scale agriculture and fossil fuel companies.[16]

Rarely is real *health* the true motivation for the adoption of these dietary fads or the marketing behind them. In fact, often the "study" that came out in the first place is funded by the industry that benefits the most from the outcome of the research.

Unfortunately, even our more traditional views of nutrition and diet have been driven by industry marketing. For instance, our obsession with protein is largely driven by the meat and supplement industry. In

16 Food and Agriculture Organisation of the United Nations, "Energy-Smart" Food for People and Climate Issue Paper," (Quebec City: FAO, 2011), http://www.fao.org/3/i2454e/i2454e.pdf

2015 the meat processing and production industry spent $4.58 million on lobbying the USDA on nutritional guidelines.[17] We can thank the surplus dairy production and subsequent government marketing campaigns post World War I for our milk and cheese cravings.[18] We use this surplus for our nauseating school lunches, supported by government subsidies. Similarly, research in the 1960s that highlighted the deleterious effects of dietary fat was bought and paid for by the sugar research foundation.[19]

The United States consumes the most sugar of any country on Earth. Even though the U.S. is the 11th wealthiest country in the world, it lags behind almost all developed economies when it comes to health. The way our culture has approached nutrition and food education simply hasn't worked. I think it's time we create a new approach that has our well-being in mind. [20]

Indigenous cultures around the world have been eating a diet that is dominantly whole grains, legumes, and vegetables for thousands of years, and yet millions of people today think grains are inherently "bad".[21]

---

17 Karlan-Mason Galen and Rebecca Shi, "The Food Pyramid & How Money Influences USDA Dietary Guidelines, " accessed May 31, 2021, https://www.greenchoicenow.com/v/food-pyramid-usda-dietary-guidelines

18 Nicola A. Hanania, Sidney Braman, Sandra G. Adams, Ruth Adewuya, Arzu Ari, JoAnn Brooks, Donald A. Mahler, Jill A. Ohar, Jay Peters, and Shahin Sanjar. "The Role of Inhalation Delivery Devices in COPD: Perspectives of Patients and Health Care Providers." *Chronic Obstructive Pulmonary Diseases: Journal of the COPD Foundation* 5, no. 2 (April 2018): 111.

19 Andy Hooke,"Cheese: A Brief History And The Origins Of Why Americans Can't Get Enough," accessed May 31, 2021. https://switch4good.org/too-much-cheese/

20 "Statista", Total Sugar Consumption Worldwide from 2009/2010 to 2021 (in Million Metric Tons), accessed August 17, 2021, https://bit.ly/3aafNqv

21 Paul Fieldhouse, *Food and Nutrition: Customs and Culture* (Berlin/Heidelberg: Springer, 2013).

I'm not here to try to convince you to be a vegetarian or to adopt any particular dietary philosophy. Dietary choices and food ethics are full of contextual intricacies. I believe that sustainable change must be intrinsically motivated. I would like to encourage you to question the "rules" and "facts" you've been told about food.

Some questions you might ask yourself:

Who is funding and economically benefiting from your belief systems?

What agencies and industries are behind the marketing?

What "phrases" do you say to yourself or others on autopilot based on cultural conditioning (i.e., "But how will I get enough protein? "There is too much fat in that." "It's not a real meal without meat.")?

2. *Finding Foods that Nourish*

I received a call from my future husband. After spending a few days with me in Los Angeles, he was flying to visit his mother in Virginia. He had just graduated college and ate a typical American diet–mostly fast food, caffeine, alcohol, and boxed foods like cereal and chips.

"Darn it, woman..." he said, "I don't know what you did, but I couldn't get myself to eat the peanuts and pretzels on the plane."

"Why?" I asked mischievously.

"I was about to open them on autopilot when a voice came into my head and asked, *what's really in the bag*? *What's Thiamin Mononitrate? How long have these been in here?*

"As I started answering my own questions," he said, "I realized it wasn't really *food* in there, it was just chemicals and empty calories, and I lost interest. Damn you!" he exclaimed, only halfway joking.

That pivotal moment changed his relationship with food forever. He never went back to unconscious eating and found a way to relate to food that feels authentic, nourishing, and ethical *to him*. Although this new frame of mind is different from most of his peers, his health and energy levels have never been better.

I am compelled to help you create a personal approach to food that is based not on what is prohibited, or what is popular in your peer groups, but what will nourish *you*. I want you to break through not just dietary fads but through the cultural conditioning that keeps you trapped in abusive habits.

All dietary trends have their truth. Each "diet" works for someone. Does it work for you? A diet heavy in whole grains could be terrible for one person, but nourishing to another. Fats and proteins are no different. Some bodies need more substance, and others need more cleansing. For some, stimulation is necessary, while for others, calmative qualities restore balance. Something that worked at one point of your life may no longer serve you.

I've seen people take on a 100-percent raw food diet while they were battling cancer. For some, this diet played an integral part in their reversal of cancer. Afterwards, the deeply cleansing qualities of a well-implemented raw food diet began to leave their bodies weak. Transitioning to a diet that emphasizes more cooked foods, foods that are easier for the body to assimilate and build strength may be a beneficial adjustment at this stage.

I see a similar trend with many who have taken on a ketogenic diet to support weight loss. The keto diet is a diet high in fat, adequate protein and low in carbohydrates that quickly convert into sugars. When the body is depleted of its sugar reserves, this causes the body to break down fat into molecules called ketones. These ketones are then circulated in the blood and become the main source of energy for many cells in the body.[22] I often see people who have had great success losing excess weight quickly on a keto diet. However, after this initial sprint, it is common for people to get depleted. People may also feel a general sense of heaviness after several months on a strict keto diet as it is composed of quite rich and heavy foods. It often benefits people at this stage to adjust their diet to include a wider range of fruits, vegetables and perhaps even small amounts of whole grains, while keeping disciplined about the quality and quantity of their food consumption.

It is also important to remember that your body is a unique system. It has a unique shape, density, and set of needs. Our minds love to compare our bodies to others – celebrities, family members, friends, and idols – and then conclude that there is something wrong with us if we don't look like them. It is vital to acknowledge, accept and learn to love the body type we are born with. Only then, can we learn to feed ourselves the food that really nourishes us.

Ask yourself:

Do I need food that is more building or cleansing? Heavier or lighter? Am I thinking about the food I am eating and where it comes from? When I think of where it comes from, am I okay with that answer?

Remember, you're not just eating the food. You're also eating your perception of the food. You can also ask yourself:

What is my diet really feeding? My fears and anxieties? Is it really nourishing me?

22 Ana Gotter, "Gallbladder Diet," accessed August 27, 2021, https://www.healthline.com/health/gallbladder-diet

When looking at a particular food, you can ask:

What are the qualities of the food? How close is this food to its purest form (is it raw, processed, dried, pasteurized, organic, genetically modified)? How long has it been sitting on the shelf?

You may explore its properties and actions, such as:

Is it hot or cold? Do I notice that it creates gas when I consume it, or does it have carminative properties (relieving of flatulence)? Does it tend to stimulate my bowels or harden them? Is it dry or moist?

Understanding the properties of food and how they relate to your constitution form the cornerstone of an Ayurvedic diet. If you would like to explore your constitution (dosha), I've included an *Ayurvedic Dosha Assessment* in the workbook section at the end of the book. While this is a good place to start on your own, I encourage you to review your findings with a qualified Ayurvedic practitioner. It's common to get misdirected in self-assessment. Often characteristics of imbalances are misperceived as qualities of our innate constitution. A professional guide will help inform you and eliminate confusion as you build new dietary habits fit for your unique body.

For instance, if I am persistently cold, I would avoid foods that have a cooling effect on the body, such as coconut products, raw vegetables, and cold liquids. Instead, a better option for me would be to choose foods that have a warming quality, such as ginger, cinnamon, soups, stews and warm teas.

If I express symptoms of excess heat – redness of the skin, acid reflux, ulcers, balding, or "hot" temperedness – then it is a good idea for me to limit foods that are hot or acidic in quality, such as hot peppers, garlic, mustard, red meat, alcohol, cheese, and tomato-based products is a good idea. It can be balancing to emphasize cooling foods such as cucumber, cilantro, fresh juices, and coconut.

If I am a person who has an impaired liver from excessive drinking, or other causative factors, it's important that I am careful not to eat too many fatty foods, especially fried foods. While fried foods are not good for anyone, they are particularly hard to digest for those who have impaired liver or gallbladder function. Instead, there are foods that help purify the liver. These include leafy green vegetables and foods high in glutathione, such as broccoli, brussels sprouts and kale. Glutathione is a compound which triggers the toxin cleansing hormones of the liver. There are many wonderful foods that are beneficial for restoring the function of the liver.

If I suffer from constipation and tend towards dryness of the skin (which often go hand-in-hand), it is advantageous to emphasize warm and moist foods and to reduce cold and dry foods. Warm food and drink encourage the channels in the body to open and flow properly. Moist foods combat systemic dryness that produces hardness of the stools. It is also important to prioritize eating plenty of high quality fats such as ghee, olive oil, and foods with natural oils like avocado, coconut, and nut butters.

The qualities and medicinal benefits of food could be a whole encyclopedia of its own. A reference book for this is *Healing with Whole Foods*, by Paul Pitchford. As a starting point, use the guidelines in the workbook section to personalize the quality of foods you take in based on your dominant constitution. If you have a specific condition or a long-standing chronic illness, it will be helpful to seek guidance to customize a food plan.

The closer you can get to checking each box below, the better:

- ☐ **Fresh**. Avoid frozen, processed, dried, and leftover food.
- ☐ **Plant heavy**. Eat a large proportion of vegetables and fruit. I recommend a 75–100% plant-based diet for the

majority of people. About 50% of each meal should consist of a diversity of vegetables. There are some cases in which animal-based fats and proteins can be effectively utilized in higher quantities.

- ☐ **Organic.**
- ☐ **Local and in-season.**
- ☐ **Warm or room temperature, generally cooked.**
- ☐ **Diverse sources of protein**. Include a variety of legumes, nuts, seeds, whole grains, vegetables, organic tofu and small amounts of organic free-range animal protein (if you choose to eat meat). The amount of protein varies per individual, based on constitution, age, digestive capacity and physical activity. There is protein in much more than you may realize.
- ☐ **Cook with appropriate digestive spices**. Using spices is rarely emphasized in modern cooking but is present in virtually all traditional cuisines. A combination of spices like cumin, coriander, fennel, basil, cardamom, cinnamon, fenugreek, ginger, turmeric etc. can be added to almost anything to help support the digestive process. This is particularly important for beans/legumes, which easily cause flatulence when cooked without appropriate spices. Each spice has a medicinal profile and can be highly targeted to various conditions and constitutions. For a list of my top 20 culinary spices, see the workbook section at the end of the book.
- ☐ **Whole grains**. Each grain has different properties. Some people do well with more grain in their diet (typically those with *vata* constitutions and certain genetic expressions), while others have a challenge digesting even small amounts of grains (those with

more *kapha* in their constitution.)

- ☐ **High quality and unrefined oils**. Use oils such as olive oil, coconut oil, and ghee (clarified butter). Avoid refined oils, vegetable oil, soybean oil, corn oil, and palm oil.
- ☐ **Natural regional mineral salts.** Rather than using table salt, use mineral salts like Hawaiian red salt, volcanic black salt, pure Himalayan pink salt, and Celtic sea salt. These have not been chemically stripped of their natural minerals and provide vital nutrients to the body when used in appropriate amounts.
- ☐ **Small quantities of unrefined sugars.** Sucanat, maple syrup, honey, jaggery, dates or coconut sugar are good options. Again, each of these have different properties that can be utilized in a personalized way. Avoid all processed sugars.

Everything beyond these guidelines is a matter of refinement to your constitution, age, condition, season, region, and digestion. Either the food you eat serves you, or it contributes to dis-ease in your body. Building a relationship with the foods that contribute to your wellness can be a fascinating and joyful process.

It is also vital to consider the timing, rhythm, and regularity of your meals. This comes under the category of *When.*

~

***When*: The timing, rhythm, and regularity of your meals**

When you consume your food influences your digestion dramatically. One of the pillars of good health is to maintain a proper rhythm of eating. The regularity of your meals directly influences your hormonal balance, your weight, your mood, your sleep, and a whole lot more.

Take a look the timing of your eating habits:

Are they consistent or erratic?

Do you snack throughout the day? Does that impact your hunger levels at mealtimes?

How soon after eating do you go to bed?

Which meal tends to be your heaviest?

Do you ever "forget to eat" or let yourself get so hungry that you get a stomach ache when you do eat?

Do you tend to eat sweets right after eating a heavy meal?

Are your meal times largely dependent on your emotional state?

Do you feed everyone else first and then yourself?

These are all impactful things to consider when looking at your relationship with food and digestion.

You may have heard the term *biorhythm*. This refers to the natural biological cycles that our bodies undergo when left to their own, natural devices. Biorhythms are seen in our sleep cycles, hormonal cycles, life cycles, appetite, elimination, cellular regeneration, and so much more. A great book to learn about biorhythms and how to harness them for optimal health is *Change Your Schedule, Change Your Life* by Dr. Suhas Kshirsagar.

An essential part of a healthy diet is to eat in accordance with your natural biorhythms. In contrast, it can wreak havoc on your digestion to eat out-of-harmony with your biorhythms can wreak havoc on your digestion, even if you eat great food!

Guidelines to consider:

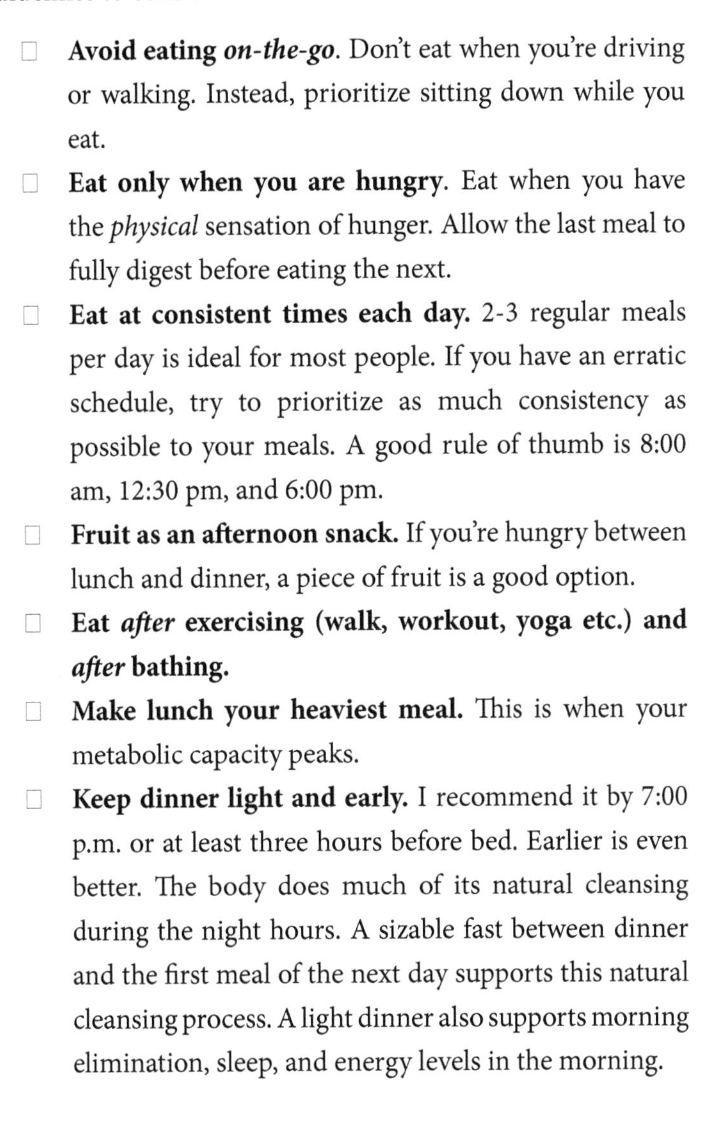

- ☐ **Avoid eating *on-the-go*.** Don't eat when you're driving or walking. Instead, prioritize sitting down while you eat.
- ☐ **Eat only when you are hungry**. Eat when you have the *physical* sensation of hunger. Allow the last meal to fully digest before eating the next.
- ☐ **Eat at consistent times each day.** 2-3 regular meals per day is ideal for most people. If you have an erratic schedule, try to prioritize as much consistency as possible to your meals. A good rule of thumb is 8:00 am, 12:30 pm, and 6:00 pm.
- ☐ **Fruit as an afternoon snack.** If you're hungry between lunch and dinner, a piece of fruit is a good option.
- ☐ **Eat *after* exercising (walk, workout, yoga etc.) and *after* bathing.**
- ☐ **Make lunch your heaviest meal.** This is when your metabolic capacity peaks.
- ☐ **Keep dinner light and early.** I recommend it by 7:00 p.m. or at least three hours before bed. Earlier is even better. The body does much of its natural cleansing during the night hours. A sizable fast between dinner and the first meal of the next day supports this natural cleansing process. A light dinner also supports morning elimination, sleep, and energy levels in the morning.

- **Avoid snacks after dinner and late-night eating**. We will talk about this more in cravings. If losing weight would be beneficial to your health, be sure to eat an early dinner and exercise before eating in the morning. Consider skipping breakfast all together, to extend the fast between dinner and the next meal.

Changing *When* habits can be a challenge because they are often deeply rooted in lifelong lifestyle habits that have been influenced by your family and culture. They can also be fueled by patterns of stress (eating on-the-go) and our typical modern work schedule (a hurried 30-minute lunch break).

While it may feel like you don't have control over *When* you have the time to eat, you actually have much more creative freedom than you might think. My recommendation is to get clear on the changes you would like to make. Then start to brainstorm creative ways to implement these changes. Even if it's not perfect at first, the experience of executing successfully on your intention is empowering and impactful!

Let's look at a couple of examples that may inspire ideas.

Vic was working in real estate. He had a nine-to-five schedule, lived alone, and was not a great cook. He suffered a long-term battle with eczema and found that his diet played a key role. Historically, he depended on either eating out for lunch or he skipped it all together. Now, he wanted to make lunch more nutritious and his main meal of the day.

He came up with a brilliant idea. He brought a stainless-steel rice cooker with a steam tray to his office. He accompanied it with some supplies like ghee, spices, lentils and rice that he could store easily in the sparsely occupied cupboards of his office kitchenette. Before he left home in the morning, he chopped some fresh vegetables like carrot, spinach, zucchini, or sweet peas. About 30 minutes before lunchtime, he took three minutes to put rice, lentils and water in the rice cooker, and drop the veggies in the steam cooker on top. Twenty minutes later, voila! He stirred in some spices and ghee, and his lunch was ready. With this simple tactic, he began to prepare fresh, warm, nutritious meals for himself while at work.

He made a variety of meals. He brought soup to warm up. He cooked noodles in the rice cooker, and made pasta or Vietnamese pho soup. He made a quinoa bowl and topped it with some roasted pumpkin seeds. Each of these meals were quick, inexpensive, and healthy!

Vic's idea inspired me and I've used it in my clinic and office spaces ever since. My clients often remark at how delicious and easy it is to make a nourishing meal. There's a recipe for *Office Kitchari* in the back of the book, inspired by Vic, which is a good place to start!

Another example – Vera typically ate dinner at 10:00 pm. She suffered from sleep and digestive troubles, for which I recommended she change her eating schedule. However, her husband did not get home from work until 9:00 p.m. on weekdays. She cooked for her husband and did not want to forgo the family tradition where they would sit down to eat together each evening. They both had busy schedules and that was one of the only times during the week they got to spend together.

Rather than accept this situation as unchangeable, she decided to cook dinner for both of them but to eat her portion in the early evening. When he got home, she offered him his dinner and enjoyed a cup of tea with him while he ate. This gave her and her husband the quality time together that they desired, and positively impacted her sleep and her digestion.

Vera's husband noticed how it benefited Vera when she ate earlier, and eventually to forge a path towards a light, early dinner while he was at work. He began to bring something to work he could heat up in the evening on his shift. When he got home, they would both enjoy connecting over a cup of tea together.

There are many creative solutions waiting to be hatched. If you say to yourself "I can't because my schedule won't allow it," or perhaps, "This person in my life won't allow it," I encourage you to take a look at the way you may *allow* others to dictate your life for you.

While there is certainly no doubt that work, family, and schedules can have a big effect on your life, we have more creative power over our lives and choices than we think. There's a strange comfort in allowing others to steer the direction of our lives. Although this gets us off the hook for taking responsibility for our own choices, it also perpetuates anxiety and stress.

Admittedly, most of my disordered eating habits were like a seesaw. On one hand, I desired control over food and my life. On the other hand, I enjoyed relinquishing control of it. I relished in both the pleasure and pain of being at the whim of something outside of myself. This seesaw contributed to my very erratic eating habits.

I find it much more fulfilling (and fun!) to make conscious choices. There are many things in life that we do not have control over. We do, however, have the ability to respond to the circumstances we are in. This is a beautiful and liberating recognition! Each decision either honors or dishonors ourselves.

As we take responsibility for our life, the rhythm, timing and regularity of our meals can take new shape – one that supports our biorhythms. *When* we eat gives *What* we eat the opportunity to move through us in an optimal way. Next, let's consider the quantity of the food we ingest.

How Much: The quantity you take in

How Much we eat is a hot and debated topic. The quantity of food that actually nourishes us depends on age, season, metabolic strength, activity, genetic factors, constitution, health condition, and the quality and type of food we eat. Do you notice a pattern yet?

How Much we eat is important and often the most emotionally charged category. We tend to attribute *How Much* we eat to how much we weigh. We often feel uncontrollable urges to eat too much, or restrict ourselves and eat too little. We commonly ricochet between these two extremes like an internal ping-pong match.

The popular calorie theory is persuasive. If you want to lose weight, intake less calories than you burn. If you want to gain weight, consume more calories than you expend. It's as simple as that. While this certainly works for many people with an average metabolic strength, and a specific goal in mind, calorie counting also has its downfalls.

First off, calorie counting doesn't take into consideration age, metabolic strength, genetic factors, constitution, and stress levels. These factors influence how food is digested, eliminated and stored in the body. This explains the dichotomy when people hopelessly exclaim "I'm eating hardly anything, but I've hardly lost any weight!" Or conversely, those who eat all day long and cannot gain a pound.

Second, learning to calorie count often initiates an addictive cycle of disordered eating. I see this particularly often in teenage girls whose early lessons in nutrition and weight, both socially and academically, center around calories. The practice quickly becomes an obsession fueled by a complex web of internal and external pressures. In a developmental period that is so vital, the cycle of obsession and depletion can be extremely harmful, physically and psychologically.

Third, calorie counting alone does not take into consideration the quality, the nutrients, and the timing of food intake. Ultimately the *What* and the *When* inform the *How Much*. It is a personal and contextual relationship.

If you're trying to lose weight, eating less can be important, but it's imperative to be paired with increasing your metabolic capacity. This includes eating the right foods, at the right times, and engaging in proper movement and exercise. It is crucial to explore why you have an appetite to consume more food than may be balanced for you.

For instance, people with obesity often have large appetites, and it's not just mental. According to Ayurveda, there is a relationship between how extra fat is stored in the body and the way heat is stored in the body. Adipose tissue acts as an insulator and can trap heat. This heat can fuel an appetite, a digestive "fire", that perpetuates the cycle of eating more and then gaining more weight. An excellent remedy for this is sweating. Sweating acts as both a form of detoxification and dispels excess heat from the body. Paired with lowering excessive food intake, this combination of actions is a powerful tool to counteract obesity. As excess heat and toxicity leaves the body, people often find that their appetite naturally lowers.

When the body is in balance it craves what keeps it in balance. When the body is out of balance, it craves what keeps it out of balance.

– Ayurvedic Proverb

If you're trying to gain weight, eating more is not always the best option. Simply taking in more calories can overload your system and create stagnation if your body cannot digest it well. It's helpful to build your appetite. Eat smaller meals more often. Encourage the growth of tissues through proper exercise. Emphasize building foods like dates, nuts, root vegetables, and "good fat" foods like avocado and ghee. Perhaps most importantly, enjoy and take pleasure in eating. We will talk more about this later.

For some, discipline around *How Much* you eat is imperative. For others, it is important to relax around *How Much* you eat. This is why it is so critical that we get to know ourselves, as the remedy for one person can damage another.

~

A few years ago, Anabel spoke to me about her challenges with her menstrual cycle. It had disappeared for months, and she didn't know why. She wanted to have children but feared she would not be able to. She felt kind of "*girlish*" without a menstrual cycle.

As we began to talk about the issue, her insecurities about her body surfaced. She was very thin and suffered from amenorrhea, the loss of menstruation. She upheld strict body standards throughout her childhood as a ballet dancer. When we spoke, her most intimate relationship felt strained and she felt disconnected from her friends and family.

I reminded her that our bodies change as we age. We are not meant to keep our teenage form. I described how some softness and curves on our bodies are healthy and important for reproduction. I pointed out how many conversations with friends in her life surrounded weight and body image, and I encouraged her to intentionally seek connection around other interests that are important and inspiring to her.

A couple of years later, she called me and shared how that conversation had changed her life. Ironically, while she struggled with not feeling *womanly*, she had been holding herself to the body image of a *girl*. She was able to gain some healthy weight by eating more freely and reframing her views about her body. She brought a beautiful baby girl into the world. In fact, she got pregnant enviously fast and had an incredible birth experience.

She had to learn how to relax and expand her *How Much*.

I know that is not the story for everyone. For others, eating less and creating discipline is important. Both overeating and undereating can create severe and long-term health conditions.

Consider that the body is made up of thousands of channels – like blood vessels, nerve pathways, connective tissues, organs, and energy meridians. These channels all co-exist and interact to make up the human body. It's similar to how a city is connected by a complex system of roads and pathways. When the roads are in good shape and can accommodate the flow of traffic, life flows well through the city. If the roads do not get the maintenance they need, they break down. If the flow of traffic is too heavy for them to accommodate, everything gets backed up, congested, and inflamed. The body is similar. With too little nourishment, our channels begin to break down. With too much, they get clogged and congested. If this goes unaddressed for a long period of time, both can create severe issues to the whole system. Our goal is to feed the body exactly what it needs to keep the tissues healthy and fuel the body with energy that can flow freely through its roads and pathways. This creates a healthy, balanced body.

While most common diets recommended calorie counting, I take a different approach. I recommend you eat until you are ¾ full. More specifically ½ full of food, ¼ full of liquid, and left with ¼ space. The stomach needs space for the digestive enzymes to churn its food. Imagine loading a laundry machine. You put in only enough clothes for the machine to handle, leaving enough space for the liquids and soaps to churn the soiled laundry. If you overload the machine, it malfunctions. So does your stomach.

When you build a real-time relationship with how much you eat, you learn to ensure the quantity you intake is manageable for your digestive organs. When you eat the proper amount of food, it prevents lethargy and helps you feel hungry by your next mealtime. If you tend to overeat, cut back to three-quarters. If you tend to undereat, then adjust your intake to three-quarters.

How much is three-quarters full? It's not a certain number of calories, nor a certain number of grams.

Imagine what it feels like, in your body, to feel really hungry. What sensations do you feel when your stomach is totally empty, only inhabited by your increasingly impatient stomach acids?

Now imagine what it feels like to be really full. What does it feel like when you can't take another bite because there is no more room?

About three-quarters of the way between those two experiences is the sweet spot: the feeling of being *satisfied*, rather than *full*. Try it next time you eat and see how it goes.

This will help you build a *sensory* relationship with your food, rather than a *mental* relationship with it. This sort of embodied relationship with your digestive organs can completely transform your relationship with food. This may take some time. Be patient with yourself as you get to know the sensations in your body.

As you do this, you may start to notice the subtleties of your appetite. Just as a mother learns to listen to the cues of a child's hunger, we can learn to listen to our body's communication. In a balanced state, it tells us when it's hungry, when it's satisfied, and even the qualities of food that it needs. As our biorhythms harmonize, this will likely take on predictable rhythms that can be accurately anticipated and built into a sustainable lifestyle.

There are general nutritional suggestions we can take such as recommended daily intake of vitamins, minerals, nutrients and calories. We can elaborate on that with Ayurvedic recommendations such as eating your heaviest meal at mid-day, enjoying a lighter dinner, and following recommendations outlined for your constitution. Ultimately, though, *How Much* to eat is a nonlinear equation. It is something you must build a personal relationship with.

It is also tied closely with our final category, *How* you eat.

~

How: The mindset and demeanor in which you eat

How we eat is the most overlooked component of healthy eating, and perhaps the most imperative. The choices we make in each of the other categories often depends on our mindset when we make those choices.

You can eat the healthiest food, but if your stomach is clenched, your breath is shallow, and your adrenaline is high, you will not digest it well.

If your body is in a *stress response*, you're not in a *digest response.* Learning to eat and make choices from a relaxed position is absolutely life changing. But how the heck do you do that?

You have likely heard of the *fight*, *flight*, or *freeze* response. It is another amazing intersystem connection found between the gut and the brain, which is controlled dominantly by a neural highway called the vagus nerve. This biological response is triggered when the *sympathetic nervous system* is activated.

The vagus nerve, also referred to as the "wandering nerve," extends from the brainstem, down the jaw, neck, and chest and connects to virtually all of our internal organs—the heart, lungs, liver, spleen, gallbladder, digestive, and reproductive organs.[23]

It is the gut-brain superhighway that sends bidirectional signals to and from the enteric nervous system (ENS) in the gut to the central nervous system (CNS) in the brain. About 90 percent of its signals travel from the ENS to the CNS or from the gut to the brain. These signals are what we call our "gut" feeling.[24]

The vagus nerve powers up our involuntary nerve center – the *parasympathetic nervous system* – and controls unconscious body functions like digestion, heart rate, breathing and our inflammatory response. The vagus nerve is now implicated in most chronic diseases such as autoimmune disorders, eating disorders, anxiety, and depression. Emotionally, it is responsible for our feeling of safety and connection in the world.[25]

When you feel endangered, by a real or perceived threat, the vagus nerve sends signals to the body and brain to activate the sympathetic response, or the *fight-flight-freeze* response. This activates virtually all systems in your body to respond to the threat: your heart rate increases, respiration becomes more rapid, and blood flows away from the vital organs and toward the periphery. Digestive function is inhibited and stress hormones like epinephrine and norepinephrine are

23 Leslie L. Klenerman, *Human Anatomy: A Very Short Introduction* (Oxford: OUP Oxford, 2015).

24 "Physiopedia," "Vagus Nerve, accessed July 2, 2021, https://www.physio-pedia.com/Vagus_Nerve

25 Tom Seymour, Tom. "Everything you Need to Know about the Vagus Nerve," accessed July 21, 2021, https://www.medicalnewstoday.com/articles/318128

secreted. This helps you to make quick decisions and transfers more blood to your muscles to help fight, run, or hide from whatever threat you've encountered.

On the contrary, the feeling of safety and connection is tied largely to the *parasympathetic* response, or the *rest and digest* response.

Without a threat present, the body and mind are able to resume their natural functions of restoration, digestion, and enjoyment. Digestive organs, like the stomach, secrete digestive enzymes. Adrenaline is inhibited, and hormones like acetylcholine are secreted to slow the heart rate and to create a feeling of serenity.[26]

The parasympathetic nervous system governs sexual arousal, salivation, lacrimation (production of tears), urination, digestion, and defecation.[27] This is interesting to look at in the context of eating habits. Most of these are directly tied to the habits, feelings, and consequences of our relationship to food. Our appetite, our digestive capacity, our bowel movements, our emotional health, and even our sensual enjoyment are connected both to our food habits and to the state of our nervous system.

The sympathetic and parasympathetic systems are both vital to a healthy human body. The ability to move between the two in appropriate circumstances is what creates tonality of the vagus nerve and general well-being.[28]

The vagus nerve thrives when it alternates between stress and relaxation in a balanced way. The ability to successfully traverse stressful

---

26"Lumen," Lumen Learning, accessed July 12, 2021, https://courses.lumenlearning.com/boundless-ap/chapter/functions-of-the-autonomic-nervous-system/

27 "Lumen," Lumen Learning, accessed July 12, 2021, https://courses.lumenlearning.com/boundless-ap/chapter/functions-of-the-autonomic-nervous-system/

28 Sigridr Breit, Aleksandra Kupferberg, Gerhard Rogler, Gregor Hasler, "Vagus Nerve as Modulator of the Brain–Gut Axis in Psychiatric and Inflammatory Disorders." *Frontiers in Psychiatry* no. 9, (March 2018): 44.

situations and then return to a calm state of mind and relaxed body creates a healthy nervous system – kind of like a gym workout for your nerves.

Most chronic disease is tied to an overly dominant *sympathetic nervous system*, in which the overworked functions of the sympathetic nervous system (the stress response) result in physical and mental imbalances.[29]

Imagine that the *parasympathetic response* of *rest and digest,* is home. We venture out into the world where there are both *real* and *perceived* threatening situations that require us to call upon our *sympathetic*, *fight-flight-freeze*, response. Even just excitement or nervousness can evoke the stress response. But we always return home, to *rest and digest*. We know where it is, how to get there, and that it's a safe and cozy place to be.

Unfortunately, most of us today live in quite the opposite reality. We spend most of our time in our *sympathetic* system, fighting off threats—be it physical or emotional. We compete for resources, worry incessantly, and drive around in our cars (a normalized life or death scenario). Most of us just try to *get by* in some way or another. It's rare to return to the *parasympathetic response* without external help like a massage, a yoga class, a vacation, a glass of wine, or whatever your parasympathetic dose of choice may be.

We feel the effects of this in various ways. In chronic stress. In the loss of our sex drive or the over-reliance on it. In chronic pain and inflammation. In dissatisfying relationships, poor sleep, or poor eating habits. All of these outcomes, over a long period of time, can lead to diagnosable disease.

---

29 Harvard Health Publishing. "Understanding the Stress Response," accessed May 17, 2021, https://www.health.harvard.edu/staying-healthy/understanding-the-stress-response

The *stress response* becomes *normal*, and *rest and digest* becomes *occasional*, or *never*. We wonder why we have a culture riddled with chronic disease, addiction, and challenges with food and digestion.

We all have unique characteristics associated with our stress response. We can move from feeling calm and grounded to angry, upset, frightened, or anxious in a moment. What we do with that stimulus is what we call our *stress response.*

The polyvagal theory outlines four categories: *fight, flight, freeze* and *immobilize. Immobilize* is an important subcategory of *freeze.*[30]

Fight is an instantaneous urge to defend yourself through verbal or physical defensive posturing. Essentially, you "fight back" when feeling threatened. This is a very effective defense mechanism when faced with a real threat if you are capable of winning the fight. It is not useful if you are ready to fight at all times, whether or not there is a real threat present.

Flight refers to the urge to quickly get away from a perceived threat – to outrun someone. If fighting back doesn't seem like an effective option, you may instead choose to flee the situation. You may physically escape, or emotionally disconnect from it. You may mentally disassociate, or intellectually redirect someone.

Freeze is the neurological response of becoming still, silent, and unseen. Evolutionarily, it is connected to our reptilian roots, literally the part of our nervous system that comes from our reptilian ancestry. Reptiles are notorious for successfully implementing the freeze response when they are threatened by a predator. They become completely still and change their colors to blend in with the environment. When faced with a frightening scenario, your most effective option of defense may

30 Stephen W. Porges and Deb Dana, *Clinical Applications of the Polyvagal Theory: The Emergence of Polyvagal-Informed Therapies (Norton Series on Interpersonal Neurobiology)* (New York: WW Norton & Company, 2018).

be to become still, silent, or try to blend into the background and not be noticed.

Immobilize is a subcategory of the freeze response, where the length and intensity of *freeze* are taken to the extreme. Reptiles will immobilize as a defense mechanism and will shut down their metabolic activity to "play dead." Just like reptiles, when our nervous system responds by *immobilizing*, our vital organs start to shut down. This is considered the most detrimental stress response to our health. It is common among people who have experienced severe and repetitive trauma.[31]

I have come to know my stress response intimately. Historically, under threat, I went to *flight*. I would immediately maneuver myself away from the situation. When things got volatile in my home growing up, I left the room to be by myself. As a young child, even my food habits reflected my flight response. I sequestered food away from the TV dinner table to dispose of it in the bathroom. As a teenager, I actually ran away from home. It was my survival mechanism, and it worked!

My secondary response to threat, if it persisted, and I couldn't "get out," was to *freeze*. I would become stiff, silent, and cold. My freeze response usually manifested in extremely volatile environments and in intense conflicts with friends and family. Fight used to be last on the defense list. I held an unconscious belief that fighting back and holding boundaries would be unsuccessful. I chose instead to be quiet or blend into the background.

As an adult, this behavior continued. I found myself avoiding conflict in my marriage, work, and community. Eventually, I became aware that my unconscious survival mechanism did not serve me or

31 'Lumen", Lumen Learning, accessed July 12, 2021, https://courses.lumenlearning.com/boundless-ap/chapter/functions-of-the-autonomic-nervous-system/

anyone else. Although a flight response might save my life if I am being robbed and need to outmaneuver the offender, it is a handicap when my partner and I are having a difficult, but important, conversation. It perpetuates a cycle of violence if I am not able to stand up for myself or another person who is mistreated.

Today, I am more confident in my ability to choose the appropriate response to a threat. I am no longer in a constant low-grade state of flight. Years of yoga, meditation, women's self-defense classes and high-pressure communication training have helped me maintain mindfulness even in the face of threatening situations. Now I *fight back* when the situation calls for it, though I notice that *flight* is still my instinctual response to danger.

Mindfulness practices help me experience my stress response somatically. *Somatic awareness* is the act of observing the relationship between the body and mind. The body expresses the patterns of the mind and spirit in fantastic ways. When you learn to notice the sensations in your body and how those sensations correspond to mental, emotional and spiritual experiences, it provides great insight into your autonomic and unconscious reactions. Once you are aware of your patterns, you have the power to change them.

Through this practice, I can recognize the physical sensations of my stress response when it takes over. My breath quickens and gets shallower. My stomach contracts. My jaw tenses. My voice rises in frequency and gets a little squeaky and fast. I lose my appetite. I often get diarrhea.

When I am going into *freeze*, I stop talking altogether. My blood-pressure drops. I get stiff and cold. As a teenager, my freeze response directly corresponded to my severely compromised digestion – I literally felt like I might die. My stress response became normalized in my daily life.

As an adult, I had to learn to speak up, hold healthy boundaries, and discern between real and perceived threats. As a reminder, the vagus nerve will activate the *sympathetic response* when your mind perceives a threat, whether it is real or not.

Perceived threat, for adults, often comes when there is a history of trauma. For instance, confrontation, whether it was productive or destructive, triggered my stress response. Years of violent verbal conflagrations with my mother taught me that conflict led to punishment and separation, rather than solution and connection. Over time, I learned that confrontation can be healthy and important. I deal with conflict compassionately and hold others in my life to the same standard.

For you, perceived threat may come in other ways. Social situations, physical touch, the opposite sex, those with different political beliefs, sexual intimacy, lack of sexual intimacy, family dynamics, dogs, strangers, authority figures – there are a million potential threats and cocktails of them. Our unconscious stress response causes us to generalize danger, based on a past experience, whether or not it is harmful in the present.

When we're children, we do not have control over our environments or many of the things that happen to us. As adults, we have the ability to discern between *real* and *perceived* threats. We also have the ability to bring ourselves back "home" to *rest and digest* once we've ventured through the trials and tribulations of life.

Getting to Know Your Stress Response: Somatic Awareness Practice

If you find the following exercise hard while reading, you can listen to a free audio recording on my website that will guide you through it – www.livewiseheal.com.

Take a moment to follow the pathway of the vagus nerve inside your body. You can use your fingers to follow the pathway. Start from the back of your head, at the top of the neck. Move toward the jaw, on both sides, to the base of the ears. Now move down the sides of the neck, toward the center of the chest, then down toward the stomach. Now let your hands broaden and spread over your abdomen. That's the pathway of the vagus nerve.

Think about a scenario that was highly stressful in your life. Allow yourself to really envision and feel what it was like to be there. Cultivate a feeling of nervousness, anxiety, or whichever emotions you felt at that time.

Notice the way your gut feels, your diaphragm, your heart rate, and your breathing. Do those sensations correspond to the pathway of the vagus nerve in your body? Do you feel the channel down your jaw, through your heart center and abdomen? Do you feel any contraction in your stomach?

How do you want to respond? What's your instinct? Do you feel like fighting, fleeing, or freezing?

When you recall the event, your body and nervous system experience it as if it were happening *now*. If you really allow yourself to get into the exercise, your body will produce the same hormones and chemical signals as when the actual event occurred. This is how unresolved or "undigested" emotions, perceptions, and traumas continue to affect the physical body for years, or decades, beyond the trauma.

Now [after you read this exercise] close your eyes and think of being with someone, or somewhere, you feel completely safe. This person, or place, may be real or not. Imagine a deep feeling of love present. If you're with a person, look lovingly into their eyes. Really picture the details of their eyes, the color, the shape, and feel their loving gaze staring back at you. It may feel awkward but do it anyway. If you're in a place, take in the experience through all of your senses. What colors are there? What smells? Which sounds are you basking in?

Now smile. Laugh. Seriously, laugh. Stay there for a moment and really enjoy it.

Notice what sensations you are experiencing in your body now. How does your stomach feel? Your chest? Your jaw? Take a slow deep breath, into your abdomen. Then, slowly exhale and open your eyes.

Congratulations! You just tonified your vagus nerve.

Throughout your day, see if you can create similar experiences with the people and places you interact with.

~

Remember, undergoing *stress* then coming back to *rest and digest* is the key to a healthy nervous system. For example, yoga practices are designed to take the body and mind through a cycle of stress and relaxation. Difficult postures are followed by periods of rest, which move you intentionally from a *sympathetic state* back to a *parasympathetic* one. The ultimate aim of yoga is to find a state of peace even during a difficult posture, and to bring this same experience into our lives off the mat.

Similarly, martial arts, certain athletic practices, and meditation teach you how to traverse challenging terrain with courage and grace. When paired with conscious breathing and practiced regularly, these crafts tonify the vagus nerve. In fact, true mastery of any of these fields requires the practitioner to achieve a high level of calmness and focus in the face of extreme pressure or competition.

There are a multitude of daily experiences that help you return to a *parasympathetic* state. The doorway is any experience that makes you feel safe and connected. Eye contact, deep breathing, meditative practices, singing, chanting, dancing, positive social relationships, laughter, massage and other forms of loving touch like a hug or enjoyable love making are all examples.

Interestingly, practices that tonify the vagus nerve have been a centerpiece of traditional and indigenous cultures globally for thousands of years. Think art, music, community gatherings and meditative arts. The wisdom of these practices is the antidote for many of the poisons of the modern age. Unfortunately, these values are often the first to be sacrificed when we bump up against our modern lifestyle.

Your Stress Response & Food

Take a moment to reflect on what your typical response is to stress.

When confronted with a threat, physical or emotional, do you tend to respond by fighting back verbally or physically? Do you look for a way to separate or escape? Do you freeze and try to blend into the background?

Think of a few recent or past examples. Your response may vary in different situations.

Now consider which character (fight, flight, or freeze) your stress response typically took on as a young person? How did you respond to your parents? To social pressures at school? To traumatic events? What kinds of foods do you go to when you're stressed? When do you eat them? How and how much do you eat?

Were your survival mechanisms effective? Your answer is most likely yes because you're here reading this book. Regardless of the intensity of your experiences, you made it.

A congratulatory exclamation for that success is a bit of a double-edged sword because the very behaviors that help you survive as a young person are likely to hold you back as an adult.

"The walls that keep us safe as children are what imprison us as adults."

I resented that saying when my mentor would say it to me. While I understood it in concept, I felt incapable of changing. The more I turned the microscope of awareness inward, the more I felt like the definition of insanity – doing the same thing over and over expecting different results. My habitual patterns of behavior left me feeling powerless, self-critical, and hopeless.

It wasn't until I started to experience the *somatic* reality of my stress response, and my conscious ability to shift it, that I began to deconstruct the walls I had built long ago. As I started to respond differently to fear and stress, my relationship to eating also changed.

Stress and eating are intimately connected. As I prepared to write this book, I did a survey of people's eating habits. A whopping 93 percent of respondents, 124 out of 135 people, said they either "stress eat" or "stress didn't eat." While that number is huge, it did not surprise me.

One of my clients wrote to me about her experience after taking the survey.

She said:

I have noticed an issue I've had with food which causes me to feel unworthy. I want to talk about it in order to release and possibly heal from it.

I feel I have used food to sabotage my relationships.

For example, I went on a date where I wasn't hungry. The man kept asking me to order food, so I ordered something small, an appetizer. Then I ate from his plate. Not out of hunger but out of nervous energy. This action turned him off.

I have noticed this is a new behavior that I have acted on in the past four years. It's one I'd like to stop.

It's funny that when I am at home, or alone, I eat normal portions until I am full. But when out with people I suddenly have uncontrollable eating. Even when I am full, I eat.

When looking back, this started with my first boyfriend whom I dated from high school through college. This was something he would do. He would order his food and somehow convince me to order what he liked so he could eat both plates.

I was thin at the time and didn't eat much so I was okay with it at first. But then I got angry because I didn't want to order what he wanted.

I also ate veggies more often than meat. He'd always order a meat dish for me because he knew I would just eat the sides. I allowed him to bully and guilt me into feeling bad for eating my own plate.

Similarly, my ex-husband always told me I wasn't good enough. Now, I seem to self-sabotage in all my relationships and make myself look greedy about food by taking more than I need in front of friends and dates. It's as if I am trying to make them reject me.

At first, I didn't understand where it came from. This morning, I had an epiphany about how my history connects to my nervous eating habits.

I see how my self-deprecating behavior corresponds to my feelings of power in relationships. I would like to create relationships where I don't feel dominated and controlled and be willing to speak to it rather than "eat it down."

Aloha,

Ana

Ana's story is an example of how her eating habits took on the character of her nervous response. It's common for people's eating habits to change drastically when stressed or anxious. In fact, it would be an anomaly if they didn't.

My stress eating habits have changed throughout my lifetime. While I consider myself to have a healthy diet and relationship with food, my eating habits still take on a different character when I am stressed. I used to binge eat. Now, I lose my appetite – I feel my stress most in my stomach. In Ayurveda, we would say my *agni* (digestive fire or metabolic capacity) lowers.

How do your eating habits change when you're stressed vs. relaxed?

In a state of stress, our energy and blood travel toward our brain and limbs so we can think and move fast. In a state of fear, our diaphragm contracts. The muscles around the stomach tighten. This inhibits our digestion, and a myriad of other physiological functions. The breath quickens and becomes shallow. Gaining control of the breath is the first step to reversing this spiral.

Change Your Breath, Change Your Life

Fred was a Jamaican drummer for my modern dance classes at the studio where I spent my evenings in high school. Outside of the studio, you could also spot him in downtown Denver on 16th Street, rhythmically serenading pedestrians for tips. He was always cheerful, a little grungy, and looked a bit stoned. Whether it be from marijuana or just the bliss of doing what he loved, I never quite knew. Maybe a combination of the two.

My dance community was dominantly African American, and full of soul! Through the people and traditions, I fell in love with African culture and dances from around the world. It was my haven away from school and from an emotionally volatile home.

During a class one evening, after I leapt and spun across the floor toward Fred at full speed, he motioned to me. He said in a very serious voice (out of character for him), "Madison, you're not breathing."

A few minutes later, on the next pass across the floor… "Breathe, Madison, breathe!"

At the time, his commentary was a bit annoying and uninvited. Yet it stuck with me like a dead bug on a windshield. I had no idea how important that gifted little piece of wisdom would become.

When I stepped into the yoga studio a decade later, my teacher told me that my breathing was shallow. As a professional dancer, I could do most of the yoga postures like a model on the cover of Yoga Journal. Breath practices were a different story. I was about as incompetent as a goldfish drinking water out of a straw.

Long, deep, abdominal breathing, especially anything that prolonged the exhale, felt nearly impossible and brought on feelings of deep and intense anxiety.

Having a history of asthma, it didn't surprise me that breathing was a weakness. I didn't know, however, how much it related to my health problems and my eating habits.

Diaphragmatic breathing, or breathing that fully engages the diaphragm for respiration, is the secret code that opens up the door to the *parasympathetic response*, the *rest and digest* response. You can also think of it as *abdominal breathing*. When you're doing it correctly, your abdomen expands on your inhale and descends on your exhale. Imagine having a balloon that grows in your belly when you inhale and deflates as you exhale.[32]

Take a moment to notice your normal, uncontrolled, breath.

How are you breathing right now?

Does your chest expand? How about your stomach?

How many seconds does an inhale take? How about an exhale?

If you noticed that your breath was primarily inflating your chest, you're not alone. If your breath took two to three seconds on both the inhale and the exhale, that's pretty typical. However normalized, both of these experiences indicate shallow breathing that is likely rooted in a long-term stress response.

Now, consciously slow and deepen your breath. If your breath is isolated to your chest, I recommend that you lie down and put your hand over your belly button. As you inhale, push your hand up toward the ceiling with your stomach as you expand it. As you exhale, let your hand float back down slowly. Elongate the exhale as long as possible.

---

32 Andy Hooke, "Cheese: A Brief History And The Origins Of Why Americans Can't Get Enough," accessed May 31, 2021, https://switch4good.org/too-much-cheese/

If you cannot do this at first, don't worry. Keep trying. It will come.

When you inhale, try to bring the breath as low down into the abdomen as possible. See if you can expand the belly all the way down to the area of your bladder, and as high up as your ribcage.

Let it all hang out – like you're pregnant!

At some point, you likely learned to "suck in your stomach" to look thin or fit. That was probably the worst advice you ever fell for.

In the yogic tradition, the practice of breathing meditation is called *pranayama. Prana* means "breath of life" or "vital energy" and *yama* means "practice of".

Yogis will work to slow and deepen their breath for years. Some work towards *one breath per minute.* That means one cycle of inhalation and exhalation lasts a full minute or longer. That's a far cry from the typical three-second breath!

If you're a singer, a diver, or a wind musician, you have probably been taught to breathe diaphragmatically. You understand the power of your breathing patterns. Calling upon these in times of stress is important for you.

Shallow breathing goes hand-in-hand with the sympathetic nervous system, the *stress response.* As you learn to consciously control your breath, by slowing and elongating it, you gain acute control of how you navigate between your *stress response* and your *rest and digest* response.

The diaphragm plays a huge role in breath control. This amazing musculotendon structure is located at the base of the ribcage. It's horizontal orientation, resembling a parachute, separates your lower vital organ chamber (the intestine, bladder, liver, spleen, etc.) from the upper chamber that houses your heart and lungs. The diaphragm is responsible for the action of respiration.

In a state of fear, or stress, the diaphragm naturally contracts, and constricts the expansiveness of breathing. It also contracts when you "suck in your stomach."

On its upper side, the diaphragm attaches directly to the pericardium, the watery sac that surrounds the heart. Therefore, the movement and rhythm of the diaphragm have a direct impact on the heart. When you breathe diaphragmatically, you are essentially massaging the heart. This stimulates circulation and oxygenation of the whole body.[33]

Not surprisingly, the vagus nerve also traces its way around the heart. It's most superficial point (closest to the surface of the body) is right at the center of the chest.

The symbiotic relationship between the heart, the vagus nerve, and the diaphragm is similar to the "three sisters" – they support each other to both survive (sympathetic) and thrive (parasympathetic).

Next time you find yourself ___________ eating (fill in the blank with stress eating, binging, not eating, eating on autopilot, or with whatever pilot is driving you that day), stop for just three seconds and observe your breathing. Simply observe it.

Is it shallow, constricted, and quick?

Once you've observed it, pause. Stop or put down whatever you were about to eat.

Do the five-count breath five times (below).

Then reassess the situation.

33 "Diaphragmatic Breathing," Cleveland Clinic, accessed June 29, 2021, https://my.clevelandclinic.org/health/articles/9445-diaphragmatic-breathing

The Five Count Breath
Pranayama

The five-count breath is one technique of many to help you change and deepen your breathing patterns. I like this breath because it can be done by almost anyone, and its integrals (the "sips") can help you feel the diaphragm and the expansiveness of your abdomen.

1. Sit or lie down in a relaxed posture.
2. Take a few normal breaths in and out of your nose without trying to change anything
3. Inhale, but this time "sip" the breath through your nose in five equal parts, pausing slightly between each sip. Expand your abdomen with each sip.
4. When you've completely filled your stomach, exhale through your nose with one even, slow breath as you count to five.
5. Repeat this five times.

This technique is simple and extremely effective. With regular practice, your ability to deepen and slow your breath will increase. You may choose to extend the length of your breathing cycle to 6 counts, 7 counts, or more as you grow more comfortable with this exercise.

For some, the abdominal muscles are so contracted that you may feel unable to do deep abdominal breathing. There are techniques that can help you. I recommend contacting a qualified practitioner who specializes in breathing practices (*pranayama*), as well as seek support with abdominal massage.

When you change your relationship with your breath, it can become a superpower. In a stressful situation, slow, deep breathing will keep you calm and level headed. You will be able to more clearly discern between a real and a perceived threat. For example, you may find that you hold your breath while you eat. As you bring awareness to your breath, you may realize the food itself is not inherently threatening. The stress response you are experiencing is a projection from past traumas. If you successfully intercept your stress response, you can consciously choose what, how and how much to eat of the food in front of you. You have the power to transform an episode of anxious eating into one that is nourishing and enjoyable. Your food, then, truly becomes sustenance.

In the event of a real threat, act on your stress response! Once you're safe, you can return to your long, deep abdominal breath to transition from *stress* back to *rest and digest*. Remember, it's important not to eat during stressful situations, or while you're in a stress response.

If you experience any anxiety driven food habits, I recommend you become conscious of slowing and deepening your breath every day. Do it as a practice when you wake up in the morning, before you check your email or look at your phone. Take three long, deep breaths between every big transition in your day – before you walk into a meeting, answer the phone, or come home from work. And... Before you start eating. Every time. Take three deep belly breaths. No one will even notice. But you will.

Engaging your relationship with both your stress-response and your breath can help you change your relationship to food. You can heal old wounds, and you can nourish yourself with a refreshed mindset.

When you invite a balanced relationship with *what, when, how* and *how much* food you consume, and begin to explore the contextual dynamics that govern *sustenance* in your life, you will begin to receive nourishment differently. The question, "*What would feel nourishing to me today*" takes on a whole new character, one rooted in a grounded relationship to your body, your mind, and your food.

Just as a contracted diaphragm constricts the function of the physiological heart, the walls we keep around our emotional heart are no different. As we learn to spend more time in a relaxed and receptive state, trusting ourselves and the journey we are on, we can engage the world with an undefended heart.

PART II
PLEASURE

Isn't it interesting that the mouth acts as both the channel for primal sustenance and a vehicle for intense sensory pleasure? These two seemingly opposing experiences are actually intimately linked.

Food is evolutionarily designed to taste good. In the case of plants, an alluring taste incentivizes humans and animals to ingest it, which in turn, encourages its procreation. Food's tantalizing properties can feed our addictions or the joy and pleasure of life. How we relate to it, and to ourselves, determines whether food becomes an uncontrollable desire or a balanced one.

Modern advances in the field of nutri-genomics show us that our genes express what we desire. Not only do nutrients and diet affect our gene expression, and vice versa, but we can actually turn on and off genetic expressions with our thoughts, emotions and feelings.[1]

Desire is a powerful force. Marketing, politics, and dogmatic belief systems constantly attempt to control it. Pleasure is often villainized as sinful. Greed, gluttony, and destructive power dynamics fuel the abuse of people, animals, ecosystems and *ourselves*. These are the shadow sides of desire – they are imbalanced expressions of the quest for personal pleasure.

On the other hand, desire can also inspire great feats of creativity, innovation, connection and expansion of consciousness. It is a fundamental and beautiful aspect of life to be celebrated.

We are about to explore the taboo topic of pleasure and how it relates to what we eat. I approach this section candidly, addressing subjects you may not have anticipated when opening a book about food. Some of it may be exciting. Some of it may be frightening. I encourage

1 Sarah Garone, "Nutrigenomics Might Be the Future of How You Eat," accessed July 3, 2021, https://www.healthline.com/health/food-nutrition/nutrigenomics-might-be-the-future-of-how-you-eat

you to use your breathing practice that we introduced in the previous section, and observe the sensations, emotions and memories that may surface with as much acceptance and curiosity as possible.

Food and the Erotic

Candace came to me to lose weight and change her relationship with eating. Her weight was at her lifetime high – over three hundred pounds. She generally knew what she aspired to eat but had a very hard time making it happen. Her attempts at disciplined eating would quickly devolve into anxious binging episodes that would leave her feeling sick and disgusted with herself.

She quickly discovered during our conversations that her relationship to food was largely tied to the shame she felt around her relationship to men, her sexuality, and her own self-worth. She had a long history of seeking out punishment from intimate partners, extreme sexual experiences, and dissatisfying romantic relationships.

Early in her life, she framed her sexual appetite and obsessions as just BDSM play. BDSM is a term used to describe aspects of sex that involve dominance, submission and control. When practiced safely, intentionally and consensually, it can foster a healthy sense of intimacy between partners. However, as Candace explored the intricacies of her health and relationship with food, she realized that her desire for punishment was not just isolated to sex play. She related to food the same way. She punished herself for her "bad deeds" with food – whatever she or someone else deemed those to be. Although she felt sick afterwards, she experienced an intense sense of pleasure during the binging episode itself, at least in the beginning. Her pleasure devolved into disassociation, a type of flight response, that left her feeling completely disconnected from her body.

Candace's experience with food mirrored her sexual experiences. It was challenging to untangle the pleasure, pain, addiction, trauma, and deeper longing that all seemed to be woven together.

Changing her relationship to eating wasn't a matter of simply adopting healthier food choices. She attempted new dietary disciplines for periods of time, but always slipped back into the same pattern. By the time she came to see me, she had been hospitalized many times and was fearful that her health had reached a breaking point. Homeless, living out of her van, and desperate for connection, her life had reached a breaking point, too.

Candace needed to dive into the motivation behind her food choices and to wade through the paradox of both the pleasure and the pain she sought through food. She needed to redefine her relationship with herself first, before she could truly address how she related to food.

I find this to be a common theme – what gets us off in the bedroom often mirrors how we *get off* with food. We can relate to this relationship either constructively or self-destructively.

Remember how I mentioned things which are "forbidden" have an eroticizing quality to me? My secret desire for the forbidden fueled my disordered eating. When I binged on foods that I deemed "bad," it gave me pleasure in secret. Yet, deep down, I believed my pleasure was inherently *shameful*, and I should ignore or hide it. The shame I felt, both related and unrelated to food, helped form a belief that I must keep my pleasure to myself. I was relating to food and pleasure self-destructively.

The forbidden is still erotic to me. Now, I'm inspired to find ways to enjoy forbidden foods. Once in a while, I treat myself to a brunch with close friends that's a little outside the bounds of my normal diet. I splurge on a meal that's a little bit "too" expensive. I can add a touch of the forbidden to the vibe of a romantic evening by sharing a delectably creamy bite of chocolate fondue with my partner.

In excess, these actions would be destructive. In moderation, they feed a happy, healthy body and life.

I no longer feel ashamed of enjoying my life, or enjoying food. The quest for pleasure evokes my creativity. I find ways to make my self-appointed selection of forbidden foods, such as French fries or chocolate pie, healthy and wholesome. I prioritize what is balancing for me, and let desire craft the beauty and frills around it. In my practice, I help people create a diet and lifestyle that supports their well-being without becoming utterly and completely boring. Diets don't work because restricting desire doesn't work.

Even the traditional Ayurvedic texts state that our goal is not to eliminate attachment and aversion, but to learn to become attached and averse to the right things.

Creation in all forms seems to illustrate this fundamental paradox – a dance between the need for sustenance and the spark of desire. For instance, the domestic task of raising a child is often the opposite of sexy, yet orgasmic pleasure plants the seed of procreation. The breasts function as a supply of milk to infants, yet are erotically iconic. The vagina serves as a canal for giving birth, yet boasts itself as an epicenter for extreme pleasure.

Similarly, creating a new business requires the spark of an innovative idea and the grit to execute on it with precision and reliability. The passion that's required to take the risk of financial and ideological failure must be balanced with the commitment to the core processes that ensure success. If a business has a great mission but ineffective operations, it often fails to succeed in the marketplace. If it sacrifices its innovative spirit merely to optimize its operations, it often fails to keep up with the evolving interest of consumers and the loyalty of employees.

Masterpieces, in all forms, channel the best of both *functionality* and *ferver*. Of *form* and *freedom*. Of *containment* and *wildness*. What better place to apply the wisdom of this primal polarity than to the masterpiece of our own life?

~

Esther Perel, a well-known relationship therapist, exquisitely explores the fundamental paradox between the need for *love* and the need for *desire* in her book *Mating in Captivity*.[2] *Love* evokes feelings of safety, comfort, stability, reciprocity, and trust. *Desire* conjures the longing for novelty, adventure, mystery, eroticism, and risk. These coexisting needs are inherently polarized, and often express contradictory forces within us.

Perel doesn't value one over the other; instead, she describes this as a *paradox to be managed* rather than *a problem to be solved*.[3]

In long-term intimate relationships, the dance of love and desire is a classic dilemma. What makes us feel safe and loved does not always correspond to what turns us on. Perhaps the initial spark burns out after a few years of enjoying domestic comforts. A deeply satisfying family life may collide with unspoken fantasies that could destroy it. A deeper commitment feels at odds with the erotic spark. Sex drive drops sharply after having kids. A high school girl is attracted to the "bad boy" yet wishes he would bring her flowers and sit with her under the stars. All of these are examples of this confusing paradigm.

2 Esther Perel, *Mating in Captivity: Reconciling the Erotic and the Domestic* (New York: HarperCollins, 2006), https://www.goodreads.com/book/show/27485.Mating_in_Captivity

3 Esther Perel, *Mating in Captivity: Reconciling the Erotic and the Domestic* (New York: HarperCollins, 2006), https://www.goodreads.com/book/show/27485.Mating_in_Captivity

Lenny, a psychotherapist I consult, told me recently that in his 30-plus years as a therapist, he has yet to see one romantic relationship in which this dilemma hasn't come up in some form or another.

How do we manage our need for stability that is routinely threatened by the burning, inconvenient spark which makes our eyes wander, our genitals swell, and sometimes even our hearts long for something we're not endowed to? Do we recognize it honestly? Do we act on it? Do we stuff it down? Do we find a way to honor both parts of us? What can we learn about ourselves in an honest observational practice?

The same conflict can arise in your job, your home, your family, and definitely with food. After all, food is our longest-term relationship! Managing this paradox of life is key to our satisfaction. Honesty, creativity, and compassion are the ingredients for success.

Food, just like intimate partners, can serve both as sustenance and as pleasure. Food can feel like a warm hug, and a luscious scent of sandalwood. It can feed our basic survival needs, and offer that delicious cherry on top.

Let's explore this more personally.

Think about your favorite "comfort food." When you imagine it, what do you experience?

Mine is mashed potatoes and gravy. When I imagine eating a warm, savory bowl of it, I feel happy, safe, and comforted. I imagine being in a cozy home space, cuddled up on the couch afterward with a book, some candles, a foot rub, and then falling asleep much earlier than culturally normative.

Now think about a food experience that turns you on, sparks you sensually.

Here's the first thing that comes to my mind: I'm being slowly fed a delicately crafted bite of dark chocolate mousse, crowned with a perfectly shaped raspberry. I'm in a dimly lit restaurant, serenaded by a handsome cellist about ten feet away, who looks strikingly similar to Hauser. If you don't know Hauser, he is a Croatian cellist. His erotic spark literally drips from his pores as he plays his classical repertoires, as if he is making love to his cello and anyone else whom he engages on stage.

Burn me at the cross if you'd like, but I love and want both of these experiences. This doesn't make me any less spiritual either. In fact, the more I have allowed myself to express the wholeness of my being, the more devotional my life has become. Truth and spirit are inseparable.

Food takes on the character of both sustenance and pleasure, whether we recognize it consciously or not. Problems arise when we suppress or overindulge in either one of these fundamental impulses.

Here are some examples of how these may show up:

Suppressing food as sustenance:

- Fasting to a point of depletion.
- Forgetting to eat or drink amidst a busy life.
- Focusing on calorie counting or working out to the exclusion of true nourishment.
- Feeding others well, but doing the bare minimum for yourself.
- Regularly ignoring signals of hunger.
- Believing to have or experiencing a scarcity of resources.

Overindulging in food as sustenance:

- Regularly overeating comfort foods.
- Always keeping extra food around, just to feel safe.

- Obsessing over the nutritional value of food, to the point that it is sometimes difficult to enjoy.
- Choosing food based on size – "the more the better."

Suppressing food as pleasure:

- Eating just to "get by."
- Consuming the same things day after day, because it's convenient.
- Fantasizing about foods you want to eat, but not allowing yourself to enjoy them.
- Avoiding your favorite foods, even in moderation, out of the fear of gaining weight.

Overindulging in food as pleasure:

- Often binging on food, alcohol, or other substances.
- Excessively using food as a reward or punishment for your successes and failures.
- Regularly overeating, and sometimes feeling like it's uncontrollable.
- Repeatedly eating things you know are harmful to your body, and having an aversion to foods that you know are good for you.
- Using food as a substitute for emotional pleasures like sweetness, connection, and intimacy.

I find it common for people with disordered eating habits to also have suppressed or hidden eroticism. Sometimes food becomes the only safe outlet for erotic pleasure. Imagine someone in a deeply unsatisfying marriage who has written off all possibility of sexual satisfaction. Food becomes their only avenue for sensual enjoyment. I also see cases where pleasure is denied altogether, in life and with food. Food is often wrapped up tightly with all sorts of fears or belief systems about pleasure. Now let's explore the connection between food and your eroticism a bit deeper.

In what ways do you most naturally experience and seek pleasure?

What are some of your erotic desires that you feel are taboo and are reluctant to admit?

What correlation do you see between the way you relate to your erotic desires and how you desire food?

Let yourself be really honest here. You don't need to act on what comes up. Just observe yourself without judgment.

Perhaps some of your desires feel like they threaten your relationships. They may feel like they contradict what you "say" you stand for, like monogamy or nonviolence. They may feel like they oppose your religion or sexual identity, like bisexual or homosexual tendencies, or even having desires at all. Your desires may seem contradictory. They may reverse what you feel your *role* in life is. For instance, you may have a desire to be pleasured and served when you spend the rest of your life as a caregiver. Or, you may have the desire to be dominated when you spend most of your day as a commander in chief.

Desire is not rational. It doesn't care much about morality. It laughs in the face of being suppressed or ignored. Despite its reputation, desire is not destined to harm or oppress. It can be channeled in ways that cultivate connection, inspire creativity, and bridge body and soul.

My honest desires often contrast my image, my role, and my sexual identity. I can understand the younger version of myself, afraid to express the depths of my innermost longings, exchanging honest expression for pleasing others and trying to fit the mold. When I withheld my desires, however, they did not vanish. Instead, I expressed them subconsciously: I binged on forbidden foods, manifested extreme physical tension in my body, and explored desires in unhealthy and unconscious ways.

For me, choosing to explore my longings, rather than hiding them, was step one. Talking about them openly with someone who felt safe was step two. Learning to integrate and enjoy the journey of bringing forward all aspects of my authentic self was step three.

While I still feel the paradox between love and desire, I enjoy the honest exploration of learning to dance with them both. My needs and desires always teach me something about myself. They also generate empathy and compassion for others who are navigating similar terrain. I enjoy crafting a life that honors all of me. I enjoy helping others do the same.

Accepting that I am an erotic being who can experience pleasure has been a fundamental part of my journey toward a healthy relationship with food. The quest for true pleasure inspires me to explore the beauty of taste, smell, texture, color, and ambiance. It has opened my eyes to how I relate to power and control, both with food and beyond it. It has emboldened me to turn pain into pleasure, mundane into magnificence.

On the other side of the spectrum, accepting my need to be loved, cared for, seen, and nourished has been critical to my journey toward healing my digestion. The daily practice of self care has created fertile soil for connective relationships, warmth, sweetness, meaningful community, and healthy discipline. Learning to accept nourishment has helped me learn to trust myself and listen to the cues of my body. It has guided me to turn food into medicine.

Knowing that I can accept and deserve sustenance and pleasure has been life-changing. When my cup of needs and desires is full, I naturally share my abundance. I become a sustainable circuit of giving and receiving, which is deeply fulfilling.

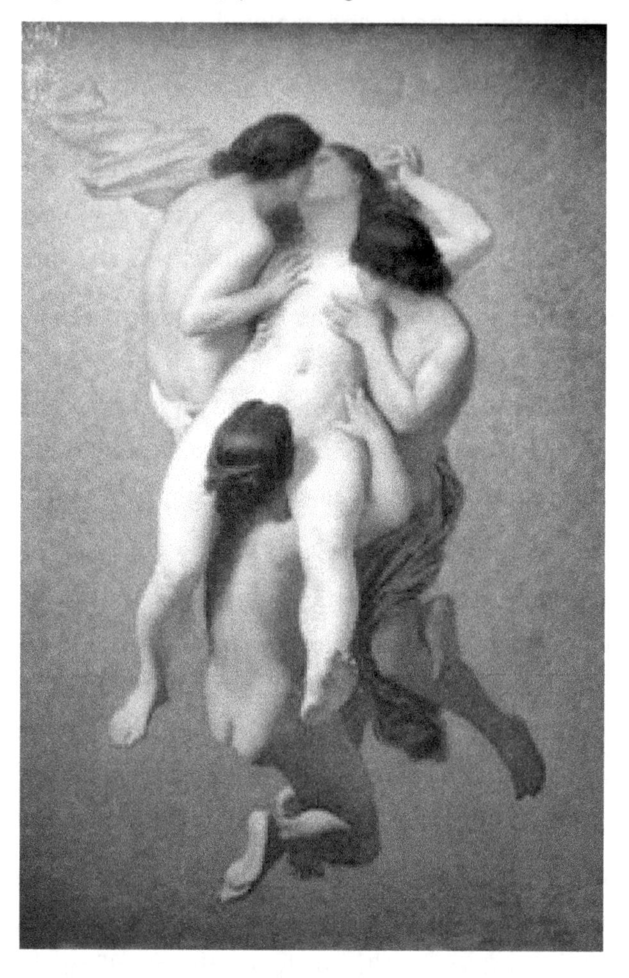

La Femme Damnée, "The Cursed Woman", by Nicolas Francois Octave - 1859

Overcoming Guilt and Shame

[For women] the very consciousness of their own nature must evoke feelings of shame.

— Saint Clement of Alexandria

Over half of the respondents that I surveyed before writing this book report that they sometimes or usually experience guilt or shame when they eat. Five percent reported always experience these emotions when eating.

As I became a self-reflecting adult, I noticed these underlying feelings which I seemed to be carrying around with me. I had never done anything horrible in my life. I didn't have any criminal desires or behaviors that made me a threat to society. So why were guilt and shame following me around?

I began to notice these feelings consistently linked to making money, having sex, holding boundaries, being ambitious, creating success, being lovable, and enjoying eating. On really bad days, I even noticed guilt and shame lurking in the feeling of being alive.

The cultural and religious narratives of the last few thousand years are laced with guilt and shame. These messages subjugate pleasure and sensuality, particularly in women and those who do not fit gender or beauty norms. I believe the unknowing internalization of these allegories is directly related to most people's relationship with food.

When I started to explore the stories and myths embedded in the fabric of our culture, I had an epiphany: I had unconsciously absorbed ideas about my identity and desires that literally made me feel bad about *who I was.* Although I did not grow up with formal religious training nor was I versed in mythology, these stories were deeply lodged in me. I did not consciously know the details and origins of the narratives that were subconsciously shaping my belief system.

Elizabeth Lesser, in her book, *Cassandra Speaks*, illuminates how the shadows of guilt and shame crept into myths like the Creation Story of Adam and Eve, the story of Pandora, and the story of Galatea (the tale of the white marble statue of the perfect woman). As a woman, these stories shaped my understanding of what it meant to be feminine.

For thousands of years, desire for anything that resembles feminine form or energy has often been considered sin. Women should feel shame for being "Woman." Men should feel shame for desiring "Woman." Go beyond the traditional gender norms of men and women, and you're bombarded with messages of shame.

Let's widen our lens of observation beyond the societal narratives of women, and examine constructed expectations of anything deemed feminine. The earth, the arts, mysticism, emotionality, sensuality, non-authoritarian leadership, intuition, herbal medicine, and beauty have all been largely labelled as "woo-woo," impractical, or dangerous.

Do the same for anything labelled traditionally masculine – work, money, war, science, rational thinking, engineering, intelligence, strength and vigor – and you'll find traits and trades that are largely thought of as acceptable, practical, and prestigious.

In yogic philosophy, as well as most other ancient wisdom practices, masculine and feminine qualities are not limited to the bodies of men and women. They are both present in all of us at all times. Creating harmony and balance between your own masculine and feminine qualities (also known as yin/yang, Shiva/Shakti, agni/soma) is key to good health and happiness. It is also the doorway to spiritual liberation. Historically, we have valued one over the other, and hence created imbalances we are living through today.

So far in the 21st century, we have begun to accept growingly inclusive gender lines and thankfully, a widening acceptance of sexual and gender identification. We have begun to break open some of the falsities and biases of religious and power doctrines that have been blindly accepted and enforced for thousands of years. People of all genders are beginning to free themselves from the prison of traditional expectations. We have even begun connecting the dots between science and mysticism. Yet, there is still resistance.

While we have a growing number of female, non-binary, and minority leaders around the world, we are still plagued with the scars of racial and gender inequalities. The United States has yet to see a female president – extraordinarily strange when you consider people with uteruses make up roughly half of the country.

Many fields outside of politics continue to carry this gender bias. Over the past 120 years, women received only 6 percent of the awarded Nobel Prizes. Explore the cache of "prized" literature throughout modern history and you will see the vast majority are authored by men – namely, white men.

Why is it that books and content written by women, LGPTIQ people or by people of color, are thought of as just content for other women, LGPTIQ people, or other people of color? (LGPTIQ is an ever growing and evolving acronym. It is an inclusive term covering people of all genders and sexualities, such as lesbian, gay, bisexual, transgender, queer, intersex, pansexual, and allies.) Whereas books and content authored by white males are generally held to be notices and doctrines for all.

Even while writing this book, I've been told that my audience will be mostly women. The unspoken expectation is that my writing, because I'm identified as a female, is only valid to other people with sexual organs that resemble mine. Why is that? This book is relevant to anyone who wants to reshape their relationship with food and themselves through the lens of it.

It's important that we expose these biases, and recognize how we hold them within us.

~

Let's return to the feeling of guilt I carried as a young woman around my desires. Because of the societal narratives that we explored, I internalized that financial security, success, ambition, pleasure, and respect were *off-limits*, *reserved for men*, or *rebellious*. My desires chafed against the role I felt I needed to play in my family and community to win friendships, get good grades, be sexually desirable, and avoid being punished or publicly shamed.

The cognitive dissonance between my desires and the role I was playing created a deep feeling of shame. I felt shame around *who I was*. Yet *who I am* is incredibly beautiful – a creative, philanthropically-minded woman who is passionate, playful, intelligent, deeply spiritual and sensually astute. My shame was attached to an underlying feeling of subordination. I felt unworthy of any feeling of power within me. These feelings led to a lack of confidence and self-repression that fueled spirals of self-criticism, dissatisfaction, and failure to create what I desired. While my self-limiting beliefs were challenging to confront, I recognized that I was actually participating in the recycling of patriarchal power dynamics that held me and others in cycles of oppression.

If you run up against a similarly mysterious foundation of guilt and shame in your life, I encourage you to look at the myths, narratives and stories that nurtured your identity. We likely share similar groundwork, athough your creation story may extend into different terrain. This may include your racial, religious, or indigenous heritage.

It is important to acknowledge that men have also been defined and repressed by the limiting belief structures of a racially biased, male-dominated society.

Nikko, a successful executive in his 30's, connected his food habits and sexuality to programmed beliefs about himself as a man by his parents, his teachers, and his role models. His hardwired beliefs equated being a man to being a macho, dominant "alpha" whose diet should mirror the cultural status quo. He was embarrassed by his desire to be a vegetarian (seen as "soft" and "weird" in his social circle) and his desire to play more of a submissive role in the bedroom (seen as "pussy" in society at large).

As he took ownership of his real desires and allowed the world to respond to his confidence, he found that he no longer felt embarrassed or ashamed of himself. Ironically, he began to feel more confident in his masculinity and his career reached new heights. While his body was white, male, heterosexual, and athletic, he embraced that his desires did not match the "norm" and actually thrived on it. He learned to communicate with openness to his partners without getting swept away or silenced by embarrassment or fear of rejection.

We each have the choice to forge new avenues of expression and connection. As we do this, we have to be careful not to perpetuate blame and separation so we may build a more inclusive and empowered global community.

"If it is a despot you would dethrone,
see first that his throne erected within you is destroyed."
- Khalil Gibran

Virtually all of the systems of power that have historically attempted to suppress desire have been de-masked in scandal. We continue to see countless cases of sexual assault from priests, youth leaders, politicians, and spiritual teachers around the world.

Suppressing desire does not work. It always seems to leak through the cracks, often in secret, painful ways that harm the very people and institutions that the religious, social, and political doctrines were meant to uphold.

According to Ayurveda, one of the primary causative factors of disease is *suppression of natural urges*. This includes hunger, thirst, urination, evacuation, sleep and sex. Withholding any of these creates imbalance in the body and mind. While uncontained desire can lead to addiction and abusive actions, natural desires all have the potential to be expressed in healthy and fulfilling ways.

Eight (Essential) Desires

Religions and spiritual practices around the world often outline desires to avoid. In Catholicism we learn of the *Seven Deadly Sins*. Yogic philosophy teaches the *Yamas* and *Niyamas*, which correspond to righteous and unrighteous actions. In Hinduism, the *Arishadvargas* outline the *six enemies* which prevent us from attaining liberation. In Buddhism, we find the *Three Root Poisons* and the *Three Pillars of Dharma*. While unique in tradition, they all express many similarities.

There is timeless wisdom to be gleaned from the practice of transforming destructive urges. There is also great value in learning to accept what I call our *essential desires*. In their loving fulfillment, we may find that they carry wise messages for our heart, and lose their grasp on our mind.

Food becomes an easy substitute in our quest to fulfill our essential desires – it often creates the experience of immediate gratification. Recognizing this, we can choose to fulfill these desires wholeheartedly, which may or may not be related to food.

Let's take a look. Below I outline eight essential desires and offer questions of reflection. Take a few minutes to notice which of these make you nod "yes" or "hmmmm maybe..."

For you, does food (or other consumable substances) relate to your desire for:

Safety and Security – Your basic survival needs like shelter, food, and money.

Do you fear that food may not always be there?

How does food relate to your financial stress?

Do you keep it around like you would savings in a bank?

Do your dietary habits resemble that of your "tribe"?

How does this serve you, or not serve you?

Connection – Your innate longing to connect and belong.

Do you reach for food when you're feeling lonely?

Do you reject or avoid food in social situations where you don't feel entirely safe and relaxed?

How do your cravings for food relate to your eroticism and your desire for pleasure?

Boundaries – Your ability to hold healthy boundaries with your body and life.

Do you let others influence your food choices?

Do you sacrifice your own desires and intentions in the face of emotional stress or external pressure?

Empathy – Your desire to see and be seen without judgment.

Do you make choices solely to impress or not disappoint others?

Do you judge yourself or others for their dietary choices? Do you feel judged for yours?

Do you consider the impact of your food choices on the people, animals, and environment around you?

Excellence – Your beliefs of self-worth and confidence.

Do you feed yourself differently when you feel successful vs. when you feel you have failed?

Do you reward or punish yourself with food or substances?

Do your eating habits feel sloppy? Are you longing for refinement?

Authentic Communication – Your ability and willingness to speak your truth.

Do you "stuff" your words down with food when you feel anxious?

Is there something that you've been holding back communicating?

Freedom – Your desire for free creative expression and play.

How does food interplay with your desire for control? Or your desire to relinquish control?

Do you feel bound?

Do your restrictive food habits mirror the way you hold yourself back from letting loose?

Is there something that your heart longs to create or express?

Purpose – A desire for meaning.

Are you longing for a sense of meaning and purpose in your life?

Do you have feelings of emptiness or uncertainty?

Does eating, or anything that you consume, temporarily relieve an uncomfortable feeling, or fill an unexplainable "hole"?

Now, I encourage you to explore:

How do your food habits play out in these scenarios?

Does food really fulfill the deeper essential longing?

How might you go about fulfilling this desire in your life, outside of food?

At the beginning of this book, I encouraged you to keep a lightheartedness to this exploration. I want to reiterate that now. Whatever feelings, memories, and emotions you feel are valid and real. They do not need to be ignored or cast aside. Nor do they need to be immediately "transformed" into something "positive."

Perhaps they just need to be looked at honestly and with a compassionate heart. They are there for a reason. Sometimes even laughing at yourself, not in a condescending way, but in a "wow that's so ironic it's amazing" kind of way, helps.

We all want to be loved. We all want to be seen. We all want to feel safe and connected. We can start by giving the empathy and compassion we long for to ourselves.

Somatic Awareness and Shadow Integration

Most of us carry guilt and shame around like a backpack. Sometimes the pack is filled with things we just picked up recently. Other times it is filled with things we've been carrying virtually our whole lives. We may even be lugging around impressions that have been imprinted genetically. For example, patterns of mass disasters and traumas, such as the Holocaust, can be traced in the epigenetic expression for generations.[4]

The big question is, how do you unpack your backpack?

You can't just put it down – otherwise you already would have, right? How many times have you vowed to change your behavior but quickly fallen back into bad habits when impulse sets in?

As you become aware of the sea of unconscious influences to your sense of identity and worth, it may feel like you are an onion peeling – layer by layer. Trying to analytically understand the forces of the past acting on your present often leads down a rabbit hole of unending mental concepts.

4 Rachel Yehuda, and Amy Lehrner, "Intergenerational Transmission of Trauma Effects: Putative Role of Epigenetic Mechanisms," *World Psychiatry* 17, no.3 (September 2018): 243-257.

What we can do is become aware of how these unconscious influences affect us moment by moment. By observing these experiences, we can create a sensory relationship with these unconscious drivers of guilt and shame. By doing so, we actually bring them to our conscious mind. A mindful, sensory observation paired with an attitude of radical self-acceptance is a powerful tool for healing.

Highly charged situations, whether they are positive or negative, are sensational. We have the opportunity to either experience the sensations or numb them. Pain and pleasure are two sides of the same coin. In fact, they activate the same part of the brain. This is why people often describe that crying and laughing create the same release.[5]

> *Take a moment to embody the feeling of nervousness or anxiety in your body.*
>
> *Notice what sensations you experience in your body and where you feel them.*
>
> *Now cultivate the feeling of excitement.*
>
> *Do the physiological feelings of nervousness and excitement feel similar?*

To me, they arouse almost identical sensations. I get a surge of electric energy that runs through me. My chest and abdomen tense a little. My stomach flutters. My teeth clench. My mind starts to spin quickly, and my legs get a little stiff and awkward.

The only difference between the feelings of *nervousness* and *excitement* is that I try to stop myself from feeling one, and revel in the feeling of the other. Butterflies and electricity shooting through my body are uncomfortable when I feel nervous. They are pleasurable in the context of excitement.

5 William Cromie, "Pleasure, Pain Activate Same Part of Brain," *The Harvard Gazette*, January 31, 2002.

This exercise is an example of a somatic approach to observational experience – becoming conscious of the sensory experiences that connect the body and mind. If you find that it's challenging for you to do this, I encourage you to continue exploring. It gets easier with practice, almost like learning a new language.

We actually speak in somatic expressions regularly without realizing it. We say things like *I'm holding the weight of the world on my shoulders*. That experience was so *jaw-dropping*. That person is so *anal*. They were so *in their head*. That person *has such a warm heart*. Or, they got *under my skin*. While we're not actually talking about the physical body, our physiological functions mirror almost perfectly the way that we express ourselves energetically.

In her book *Existential Kink*, Carolyn Elliot cuts through the psychology of changing habits by taking a sensational approach. She helps her readers recognize that we actually *get off* on the things we *think* we hate. Why? Because our unconscious always gets what it wants.

I had to recognize the pleasure I received from my unhealthy binge-eating episodes before I could change them. Similarly, realizing we actually get something from our backpack of guilt and shame is an important step. I know that might sound strange, but let me explain.

I'll never forget when I did the exercise that Carolyn outlines in *Existential Kink*. At first, I was a bit skeptical. It sounded a little like new-age jargon to me. But I followed the prompt.

After dropping into a state of relaxation and self-observation, I thought about a deeply unsatisfying relationship dynamic I supposedly hated in my life. Meanwhile, I observed the *sensations* I felt *in my body*. Where and what do I feel? Anything in my head, my heart, my stomach, my genitals?

I felt this wave of heat that started in my pelvis and rose up through my stomach and chest, into my face and head. I became aware of the tension this situation created and how much energy was pulsing through me as I related to it – even just in thought!

Unexpectedly, as I allowed myself to really feel the fullness of this energy, I just about had an orgasm – no joke – thinking about this scenario I supposedly hated! By the way, the relationship dynamic had nothing to do with a sexual partner.

This dramatic and undeniable experience was eye-opening. I knew that I now had the choice to continue relating to this relationship as unsatisfying, or allow myself to feel the energy and pleasure I actually got from it. As I invited the sensational reality of this uncomfortable experience, the relationship dynamic I was suffering from completely changed. Within days, my interactions with this person went from fearful and contracted to confident and present. I went from feeling dominated and chastised to feeling seen and respected.

This moment changed my life forever. I found I could also apply this exercise in any uncomfortable situation. Rather than trying to push away the discomfort, I could invite and even enjoy the sensational experience of it. In doing so, I allow energy to move through me freely without either clinging to or rejecting it.

This type of work is often referred to as *shadow integration*. When I realized I unconsciously "liked" the things I thought I hated in myself and others, I felt powerful. I realized my unconscious mind really does get exactly what it wants in order to perpetuate its worldview. I really am the creator of my reality. Then I wondered, what experiences could I create if my conscious mind and unconscious mind were aligned?

After years of studying yoga, it was off the mat and outside the studio that I really began to understand what yoga really meant.

The word Yoga means *union* – union with your higher self or with the greater power. The word *Guru* means to move from darkness to light, or to bring your subconscious mind to consciousness. While rare to find, a true guru is a teacher who helps you merge your subconscious and consciousness so you can experience a direct connection to the divine. Yoga helps the practitioner see their authentic self, and ultimately see themself reflected in all.

As I began to practice this shadow integration, yoga shifted from something I did to someone I was. I found life became deeply pleasurable. I could experience pleasure, not just in secret, but in broad daylight, in many forms. I discovered that the true experience of pleasure reaches much farther than just sexual satisfaction.

One of my heroes, Joseph Campbell, timelessly professes, "Follow your bliss." For me, his animated voice is like sunlight that seeps into a dark room where guilt and shame reside. Following your bliss is allowing true pleasure to light up your body and life. It is not a fleeting experience of excitement to chase. Nor is it the embodiment of evil. It's joy. It's surrender. It is following the spark of inspiration that exists within you – spark that is guided by spirit.

When I allow pleasure to flow through me freely, my experience of every aspect of my life changes. My relationships, my body, my confidence, my purpose, my spiritual practice and my life with food enliven.

When I allow myself to truly enjoy food, I finally appreciate the abundance around me – I don't need to scavenge for my next meal. I experience pleasure while eating without feeling shame or guilt. I trust my body to communicate what it needs and what it doesn't.

When I approach food through the lens of pleasure I participate in a relationship with the feeling of satisfaction. The habit of overeating naturally washes away, as does any desire to restrict myself.

"We must let go of the life we have planned, so as to accept the one that is waiting for us. Find a place inside where there's joy, and the joy will burn out the pain."
– Joseph Campbell

Getting Beyond Your Weight

In a research campaign called "The Real Truth About Beauty: Revisited," which was sponsored by Dove, only four percent of women around the world consider themselves beautiful. Ninety-two percent of teen girls would like to change something about how they look with body weight ranking the highest.[6]

Weight obsession, body image shame, and body dysmorphia are painful and challenging experiences. I am in no way trying to minimize their complexity here, but I do want to illustrate and encourage a life beyond the confines of it.

Our morphing landscape of idealized form, for all genders, is pointless. Think about how many industries would go out of business if girls and women felt good about themselves and their body. Add all others on the spectrum of gender identity, and we've got a whole different economic and cultural reality.

---

6 Joni Richards, Laurel Dicus, Sarah Drexler, Anna-Claire Gibson, and Caleigh Lentz, "Case Study of the Dove for Real Beauty Campaign," PRCM3050. https://en.calameo.com/books/00337511237b2e84ea999

Throughout time we've gone through different social idealizations of bodies. Small hips, curvy hips, big butts, small butts, large breasts, slender shoulders, big muscles, defined jawline, long legs, toned abs... Sound familiar? How many times have you compared yourself to whatever version of the idealized form you've adopted? What would life be like if you accepted yourself, as you are, as you were meant to be? If that made you squirm a bit, notice that.

Your idealized weight is likely not your healthy weight. You may have an image about what you think you should look like – what you should weigh – that's based on some social or mental concept.

As mentioned earlier, Ayurveda outlines three *doshas*. Doshas are bio-elemental functions which everything in nature is built upon – *vata*, *pitta*, and *kapha*. Each person has a combination of all three, but in varying proportions. This is what forms a unique constitution, called *prakruti*. This is kind of like a recipe. The closer you stay to your constitutional balance, the healthier you are. The farther you get from this balance, the more prone to illness you will be.

Are you naturally more curvy? Do you build muscle extremely easily? If you stop exercising, does your body rapidly shrink in mass? All of these are indicative of your natural constitution. (Reminder: If you'd like to explore your constitution, there is an Ayurvedic Body Constitution Assessment in the Workbook section at the back of the book).

When you finally accept your body's natural constitutional qualities, weight takes on a new meaning. A diet, exercise and rest regimen that is good for you may be imbalancing for someone else. Losing 10 pounds for one person could be a phenomenal improvement to their health, whereas losing 10 pounds for you could be extremely depleting and set you up for many chronic health problems as you age.

When I got honest with myself about my body image issues, and talked about them out loud, I found it kind of comical. I paid the most attention to the parts of my body I was most insecure about. My two victims were my stomach and upper arms. I thought the pudge on my lower belly made me look fat, and I was constantly trying to either suck it in or hide it. I thought my somewhat unusually muscular upper arms and shoulders made me look "unfeminine" and "bulky." I wore clothes to hide them.

I had severe stomach and digestive pain, paired with a belly-button piercing to spruce up my otherwise unsatisfactory-feeling midriff. I also suffered from nerve pain that radiated down my arms, and held unconscious tension in my arms and hands. My physical maladies matched my emotional insecurities.

In my practice, I find that it isn't until someone abandons their idea of what their weight *should be* that they discover what their healthy weight actually is. Only then can they successfully find their way to it.

While comparative thinking and goal-oriented weight programs are tempting, they usually reinforce self-destructive patterns. We usually end up feeling worse about ourselves than we did before the comparative goal. Accepting our bodies as they are today, with all of their beauty and scars, is the single most important step.

Coming from a place of radical self-acceptance is where we discover our inspiration to create a lifestyle that truly serves our well-being. Balanced weight becomes a symptom of a life built on a foundation of compassionate self-care.

Here, our physical form becomes a tool for the expression and execution of our life's work – our interests, pleasures, pains, and joys. Keeping our bodies balanced, rather than idealized, becomes the priority. Food becomes one of the tools we can use to maintain balance.

As I peeled away the layers of "idealized" imprinting, and accepted myself as I was, I felt more beautiful. I began to focus instead on my strengths and passions. I started to perceive how I felt, rather than how I looked. As I healed my emotional insecurities, the patterns of tension in my physical body also healed.

Moving from "How I Look" to "How I Feel"

What is generally most attractive about people is their confidence. That's why one person walking down the street wearing a blue bow tie and polka-dotted boxers can look extremely awkward, and someone else wearing the same thing can be oddly alluring. It's not actually what they "look like" in what they are wearing, it's how they "feel" in what they're wearing. That embodied confidence translates to a feeling in us, whether it's conscious or unconscious.

Judging the way you "look" is inherently comparative. Observing the way you "feel" is inherently experiential. This is one of the most important transformations for someone looking to change their relationship to food and body image.

When we judge the way we "look" we are often trying to perceive ourselves the way we expect someone else to see us. For example, when you look in the mirror before going out on a date, you are typically "looking" at yourself the way you perceive your date is going to look at you. I hate to break it to you, but chances are what you imagine them thinking about you is wrong.

When you go to a job interview, you do yourself up in a way you think is appropriate in the eyes of your interviewer. While there is certainly some truth to certain trends of professionalism, the confidence and ease of your projection is what will either make or break an interview. If you project yourself as something you're not and get the job, you're setting yourself and your new employer up for dissatisfaction. If you project yourself authentically and professionally, and it's a good match, you're much more likely to create a satisfying relationship. Authenticity paves the way to harmonious relationships.

When you live through the perception of how you feel rather than how you look, you invite a whole orchestra of sensations into your reality. You start to notice how your stomach feels when you spend time with certain people, and how your throat constricts when you speak about certain topics. You begin to notice things that turn you on and off sensually and creatively. You perceive how certain foods make you feel, and learn to use your own discernment about when you're hungry and what you digest well. You will begin to ask yourself how a food makes you feel, rather than how many calories it has.

For those of us who have spent time in the "body-hating" ballpark, inviting experiences of pleasure and joy are both imperative and terrifying. I'm talking about that raw, physical, sensational pleasure, the kind that makes you throw your arms open and let out an exhale of complete satisfaction. It comes in infinite forms.

Imagine the pleasure of getting dressed and loving the feeling of silk fabric on your skin. The ease you feel as your body moves freely and confidently while you meander through a playful day with your friends. Instead of looking at yourself in the shop windows as you pass by, you enjoy great conversation as the cool wind caresses your hair.

Later at home, you perceive the smell of each subtle aroma as you sizzle and sauté your favorite herbs and spices. You feel your mouth salivate and your stomach grumble impatiently. You delight in making your stomach wait until the perfectly browned bite is worthy of its delicate and boldly flavorful entrance into your warmed and readied mouth. Tenderly, you savor the experience as your head and neck melt softly backward.

Notice the here-and-now sensations and feelings in the language of each of these descriptives. In these examples, you are allowing pleasure in many forms. You are also inviting new dynamics into your life with a strong, embodied presence.

Honor the Craving, Change the Substance

I often speak to clients dealing with an imbalanced craving for sweets. They describe it as an uncontrollable force that takes over their body and mind after the sun goes down.

I usually start with this question: "Are you craving sweetness *in your life*?" denoting a meaning of *sweetness* that goes beyond food.

They virtually always look at me slightly stunned and confused. They look away momentarily, then deeply into my eyes and say, "Well… yes, I guess I am."

I talk to them about their food and lifestyle habits and solutions around them. Then we delve into how they are experiencing their personal life, the relationship with their spouse, kids, and work.

I find that food cravings directly relate to emotional cravings in some way. Recognizing and honoring the emotional cravings is an essential ingredient to successfully changing your relationship with food.

The food craving that corresponds with the emotional craving typically creates imbalance, especially in excess. Eating an abundance of sugary food as a nightcap for years is going to lead to disease. The same is true with anxiety induced binge eating or someone who turns to alcohol to escape from a dissatisfying personal life.

When you notice yourself using food to fill a role it's not designed to fill, it's time to address the real desire behind the craving. The craving is just a messenger, asking you to examine something unfulfilled in your life, something deep down you need to shift. Emotional cravings will likely express themselves in different ways depending on your constitution. People who are carrying excess weight often crave heavy and dense things like donuts and ice cream. People who naturally run "hot" fuel inflammatory conditions and emotions with cravings for spicy and acidic foods. Those who tend toward depletion and dryness often crave things like salad and dry crackers – "crunchy, munchy, dry." Their eating habits reinforce the issues they are experiencing physically and emotionally.

To heal these cycles of cravings, I like to take an integrative approach that seeks to fulfill the emotional craving while creating balance through the physical qualities of food.

Again, the craving is a messenger. Just like diets don't work, ignoring cravings doesn't work either. We've all experienced the attempted suppression of something we crave. It goes something like this:

> **Craving:** Yessss. I know you want me. Look how tantalizing I am.
>
> **You:** Oh yes, dear, I do. But no… I can't. I shouldn't. I know if I do, I'll –
> **Craving:** Yes, but I'll comfort you. I'll help you fill that hole you're feeling inside. I'll make you feel better. Don't worry.
>
> **You:** You will? No! Stop it! You're playing mind games with me.
>
> **Craving:** Fine. If you don't believe me, I'll just stay quiet and show you how much you want me by infiltrating every practical thing you do today.

… You make a healthy breakfast but fantasize about the craving.

… You drive to work and every street sign reads "Craving, this way."

…Your boss walks in and tells you how the project you were working on for the last two weeks needs to be revised by 9:30 a.m.

"That's the last straw, I've had enough, give me my f***ing craving NOW!"

The craving's influence on your mind intensifies until it's no longer bearable. You either numb out or give in.

How can you honor the craving and make it nourishing? I like to say: *Honor the craving, change the substance.*

For instance, let's talk about coffee. While phenomenally delicious and not inherently *bad*, its combination of acidity, caffeination, and vitamin depleting qualities is imbalancing for many. The short-term energy boost and subsequent crash often do more harm than good. I equate it to the difference between fossil fuels and renewable energy. Substances that give us short-term energy boosts call upon our energy reserves. Adrenaline, for example, is like voltage in an electrical circuit that is biologically designed to give us short, intense bursts of hormones and energy when we are threatened or endangered. When coffee is overconsumed, it leads to a depletion of our vitality and other unintended health issues. This is similar to the overuse of fossil fuels, which creates catastrophic externalities for the planet. True vitality, on the other hand, is not fueled by adrenaline. Just like sources of renewable energy, we each have a circuit of renewable lifeforce that we can utilize to create a healthy and sustainable life.

I've learned that people not only love the taste and smell of coffee, but they also love the ritual of it. We live in a culture where ritual is sparse.[7] It's a beautiful and understandable thing to want. When someone wants to get off coffee, I help them find something that honors the qualities they love but replaces the substance.

I've done this with virtually my whole diet. I've found a way to make all of the things I love healthy and nourishing, including chocolate snacks, mashed potatoes, macaroni and cheese, fettuccini alfredo, milkshakes, and even pies. It's become a fun challenge for me rather than an inconvenience. I use whole food ingredients and combinations that work well for my body. I look for alternatives to ingredients that put my body out-of-balance and instead find ingredients that make my meals and treats healthy *and* delicious. You can, too. I've included a common food-substitution list in the back of the book for some ideas to reference.

Changing food habits can be hard - it requires the right combination of inspiration and discipline. After sustained effort, however, cravings actually change. As your system begins to rebalance, you begin to crave the things that are balancing for you. Physiologically, different microorganisms make a home in your gut, and begin sending new messages to your brain via your vagus nerve of what to crave. Awareness of your cravings becomes a prime example of how to transform pleasure from a self-destructive force to a constructive one!

Challenge:

Think of one of your all-time favorite meals. Now, consider which components of this meal do not serve you. Perhaps it's too carb-heavy, too spicy, or the cream and cheese (while absolutely delicious) leaves you feeling heavy, congested and lethargic. Now, consider what qualities of

---

7 Gavin Wren, "The Ritual of Coffee," accessed February 7, 2021, https://brainfood-studio.com/writing/ritual-of-coffee/

food would be healthful for you. Lighter? More vegetables? Avoiding sugar or dairy? Less salt? How could you adapt the recipe to make it great for you? Your task is to make this meal totally and completely nourishing and delicious … using all whole-food ingredients.

Moving From Should to Could

How much of your life is filled with the s-word? *Should.* "I'd like to do that, but I should do this because it's more practical," "I'd like to eat that, but I should eat this because I've been told this is what's good for me," "I would do what I love, but I should do this because it makes me more money."

There is an opportunity cost to every choice. Our choice is whether we sacrifice the *should* or the *could.* When we find ourselves incessantly making *should* choices, it is a signal we are acting, and therefore, creating our lives from a position of guilt and obligation.

Most likely our actions around food will then be largely tied to similar energies – guilt, obligation, then perhaps, the aftermath of that – longing, resentment, shame, temptation.

By sacrificing the *could*, we are sacrificing our very own creative potential and fulfillment!

When it comes to your relationship with food, how much of your communication revolves around *should* and *should-nots*?

I am not necessarily advocating for you to throw caution to the wind and abandon all your practical commitments. What I am advocating for you to do is transform the "but I should" to "so I could."

From:

I really would like to enjoy cake with everyone tonight at Sara's birthday party. I shouldn't because I am trying to lose 10 pounds, and if I start, I won't be able to stop.

To:

I would really like to enjoy this cake with everyone tonight at Sara's birthday party, so I could offer to bring the cake, make it with super healthy ingredients, and enjoy a small piece. I'll be more interested to know how everyone likes the cake than I am with my own piece of it!

Should is a passive voice. *Could* stimulates a creative, empowered voice to offer solutions and options to our aspirations. This may seem like a rudimentary matter, but it can completely transform your relationship with food and beyond.

The Voice and Food

Sarah was a young woman in her late 20s. She was tall, beautiful, had a radiant face, an incredibly kind demeanor, and was about a hundred pounds overweight.

She told me how she started to put on weight after she was sexually molested as a teenager – twice. She described her younger self as thin and extremely attractive, but her sexual trauma triggered excessive eating and weight gain. She recognized that she had been attempting to make herself unattractive to potential sexual predators. She viewed "thinness" as attractive.

Her motivation remained a subconscious one until our conversation. As we talked, she began connecting the dots. She had never spoken about these incidents before, they had remained stored inside of her. She was able to communicate honestly and openly to me, but most importantly, to herself. Along with changing her eating and self-care practices, she began to focus on creating boundaries and expressing herself openly, rather than using food and weight as a defense mechanism.

We talked about how the mouth is both an erogenous zone and a gateway for nourishment. It also serves another essential purpose in our lives – *vocal expression.*

We speak. We yell. We sing. We express ourselves professionally, personally, and creatively – All through words that vibrate gracefully, or sometimes not so gracefully, from our tongues and lips.

Our mouth is not just where we take things *in*, it is also where we allow things *out*.

When I observed the connection between my anxiety and my food habits, I noticed that I often anxiously ate in social situations to avoid the discomfort of awkward communication. Sometimes I felt insecure that I didn't know the *right* thing to say; other times I felt what I *really* wanted to say was not going to be received well by my audience.

The result: I literally and figuratively stuffed my words right back where they came from. I essentially became vocally constipated. It is no surprise to me now that I suffered from pain in my neck region and often held tension in my jaw.

My experience is not unique. When I meet a client with habits of stress eating I will often ask, "What do you have to say that you're not saying?"

The ensuing conversation usually leads to places that are challenging to talk about and relationship dynamics that feel scary to address. Speaking up may require confronting a power dynamic that is unsatisfying but also provides some semblance of safety. It is frightening to speak truthfully when our social or financial security is on the line. The gems that are found in the caves of ourselves are very important. They often store brilliant ideas, but can run the risk of destabilizing a way of life that is familiar.

Fear of expressing our vulnerabilities, insecurities, and true desires can lead us to hold back our voice. This is often layered with childhood experiences of being punished in some way for speaking up, or expressing ourself in ways that deviate from familial or social expectations.

The voice is a powerful tool for connection and creation. It can be extremely satisfying, even pleasurable, to unlock.

If you relate to any of these experiences, I encourage you to bring vocal practices such as singing or chanting into your everyday life. Sing in the shower – however you sound! Sing along to your favorite songs when you're driving. Include a vocal practice in a *sadhana* (daily devotional practice), such as mantra, scripture, or song. As you practice, feel the connection between your naval point (belly button) and your voice. Sing or chant using your abdomen, just like your breath. Allow your voice to be free without trying to sound a certain way, and let yourself really enjoy the experience. Focus on the way it feels rather than the way it sounds.

If you notice yourself holding back when you communicate, find a way to express yourself in a way that feels safe and satisfying. This could be a vocal expression or a written one. Create an intention to free the words and ideas inside yourself. If you become self-conscious and aware of holding back, then commit to finding an avenue of expression.

It's possible to use our voice too much. If you often get feedback that you talk more than you listen, or impulsively lash out to the detriment of yourself or others, I recommend intentionally seeking out a space of silence. Prolonged periods of silence, while perhaps uncomfortable at first, can help you re-engage your authentic inner voice and open up to deeper listening. This could be an intentional period of silence you practice every day, or a silent retreat space where you spend a prolonged period of time. This is also a helpful practice for anyone who would like to deepen their relationship to their mind and spirit.

If you notice yourself eating anxiously, pause. Put the food down. Take a few slow, deep abdominal breaths. Ask yourself, what is it that I would like to express here? Then, consciously choose how you would like to communicate.

~

I find it fascinating that in the common translation of the Creation Story of Adam and Eve, the chosen symbol of the serpent's seduction of Eve is literally food – fresh fruit from a fruit tree! Eve, the archetypal woman, is punished for eternity for following her desires. While I understand that myth is not to be taken literally, I also recognize the messages of shame that these stories can fuel.

Apples and the sweet nectars of Mother Earth are not evil. Desire is a natural part of life that can be celebrated and channeled with discernment and creativity. Pleasure is good. It can be felt by the whole body and every sensory organ. It feeds joy and connection when engaged with a kind heart.

Women do not represent primordial sin.

Breaking cultural norms and cycles of abuse in the pursuit of truth and compassion is beautiful.

Food is good.

In case no one has told you recently, or you have not told yourself, you are enough. You are worthy of pursuing your heart's desires, being successful, and making an impact. You are lovable. You can be a leader. Your ideas matter. Your emotions are valid. You are absolutely precious!

PART III

THE OFFERING

We have one hand to feed ourselves,

and one hand to feed another.

I noticed their detached or anxious demeanors transform after just a few minutes of digging holes, uprooting weeds, and harvesting ripe vegetables. Sometimes I would catch them sneaking a bite of a shining strawberry or a sweet sugar snap pea. As if they needed to sneak anything – we all knew nature's bounty was one of the perks of having an office amidst a food forest.

I was impressed by these youth volunteers, labelled as *at-risk youth,* who came to our student farm. Their heartfelt presence and keen interest in learning touched me as we worked in the dirt together. They always left the garden bright and inspired.

These teenagers had a history of drug use, homelessness, or domestic violence and often struggled in school as a consequence. They would regularly tell me how working in the garden together gave them a new sense of direction and purpose. It mysteriously made them want to eat healthier, and they found new inspiration to pursue other opportunities to cultivate food.

When I first dug my own hands into the dirt in pursuit of knowledge and healing, I did not know people around the globe had been documenting the therapeutic benefits of gardening for decades. I also didn't know horticulture therapy was an academically proven modality. Its scope includes rehabilitation of mental health conditions, PTSD for war veterans, physical rehabilitation, and reformation of distressed communities.

The inspiring stories of my volunteers are a sample among thousands. In many of our large metropolitan cities, urban food forests have been built to give poor communities access to fresh produce and a personal relationship with nature. Similar projects have combined urban gardening with housing projects, creating vocational training and paid jobs for homeless communities.

A trainee at the Homeless Garden Project in Santa Cruz, California stated, "Almost every single job involved in gardening has a lesson to teach – a life lesson. From seeding and watering in the greenhouse, you learn that attention to detail is so important. Life or death for those little seeds depends on your continual watch and care. When you watch the plants grow and grow and bloom – somewhere inside, you are growing and blooming, too. This begins a foundation of self-worth and respect."[1]

My first experience with abundance came from the community garden – an abundance of food, beauty, knowledge, and community support. It offered me an incredible experience of growth and fulfillment. Simultaneously, my hard work offered hundreds of people fresh fruit, vegetables, herbs and spices. The amount of food three women and a handful of occasional volunteers can grow in just a few months is extraordinary.

The cumulative wealth of community gardening cultivates virtually all of the qualities to support the tonified vagus nerve we discussed in Part I.[2] It encourages positive social relationships, a sense of purpose, the relaxing effect of being in nature, physicality and movement, and resource abundance. It creates a sensory-rich, first-hand experience of the true essence of food – the life cycle, interdependence, delicacy, and its innumerable *offerings*.

---

1 Lee Erica Elder, "Green Thumbs Up," Institute for Children, Poverty & Homelessness, ttps://www.icphusa.org/wp-content/uploads/2015/01/ICPH_UNCENSORED_3.2_Sum mer2012_GreenThumbsUp.pdf

2 "Nature Knows Best: What is The Vagus Nerve?!," Sapulpa Times, accessed 3 March, 2021, https://sapulpatimes.com/nature-knows-best-what-is-the-vagus-nerve/

Food is not just taken *in* by us, but it is given *out* in many forms.

Food is grown, harvested, and distributed. Meals are cooked and presented. Mother's milk is nursed to infants. Goodies are fed to children and guests. Delicacies are enjoyed by lovers in sensual exchange. Bread is broken at holidays and given to those less fortunate. Food's bounty is offered by nature ad infinitum. It is excreted in actions of purification, and what's left is eventually given back to nature to be eaten by another species, decomposed, and recomposed to provide nutrients for food to come.

It is no coincidence that food overlaps so often with the act of giving and sharing.

In countries like India and Tonga, offering food is one of the most fundamental and valued parts of life and relationships. Cooking for someone or feeding a guest is not an obligation. It is a joy, an honor, an *offering*. It is an invitation for communion.

The United States, by contrast, has an impersonal grab-and-go culture around food. Unsurprisingly, western culture boasts itself more on efficiency and financial success than on the value of service and relationships.

As I write this, I am sitting in Austin, Texas, amidst the novel 2021 winter storm which left millions without power and clean water. I am fortunate to be in a home that shares power with a hospital, considered an essential service, but nonetheless lost access to clean water. The surrounding water treatment plants went down as Texas implemented rolling blackouts to stave off total electric grid collapse. Texas, the Lone Star State, prides itself on its autonomous utility grid that, for many years, boosted the local economy by keeping energy supply and demand within the state. However, when unexpected extreme weather strikes,

Texas cannot rely on its neighboring states to borrow power. Its radical autonomy short-circuited its relationship with its community.[3]

In America, we've been living in a culture that values autonomy over communion for generations at the expense of critical pillars of human health and happiness.

America's Loneliness Epidemic is a perfect example.[4]

In a 2019 nationwide study, Cigna surveyed more than 20,000 adults utilizing UCLA's Loneliness Scale. The global health services company found that 43 percent of respondents sometimes or always feel lonely, isolated from others, and their relationships are not meaningful. Another 27 percent rarely or never feel as though there are people who really understand and connect with them.[5]

The Loneliness scores were highest (most lonely) among the younger generations with the youngest generation, Gen Z, feeling the loneliest.[6]

The researchers attribute the figures to the current lifestyle trends of Americans. More people are focusing on work, living farther away from loved ones, and relying on social media interactions as opposed to face-to-face relationships. Rising economic pressure,

3 Garrett T. Galvin, "Lone Star Colar: Challenges and Opportunities in Post-blackout Texas," California: JDSUPRA, 2021, https://www.jdsupra.com/legalnews/lone-star-solar-challenges-and-8224877/

4 Susie Demarinis,"Loneliness at Epidemic Levels in America," Explore 16, no. 5 (September-October 2020): 278.

5 Jena Hilliard, "Study Reveals Gen Z as the Loneliest Generation in America," Addiction Center. accessed May 22, 2021, https://www.addictioncenter.com/news/2019/08/gen-z-loneliest-generation/

6 Jena Hilliard, "Study Reveals Gen Z as the Loneliest Generation in America," Addiction Center. accessed May 22, 2021, https://www.addictioncenter.com/news/2019/08/gen-z-loneliest-generation/

existential threats like climate change, and more difficulty starting a family also contributed.[7]

As a society, we are experiencing a true lack of connection. An incredible amount of people are suffering from stress and loneliness driven food habits, as feelings of safety and connection are tied directly to health and food. We seem to be rapidly losing connection with nature, with each other, and with ourselves.

~

As I pondered this section of *food as an offering*, I took a walk with my sweet husky-shepherd, Shyla, to the dog park. Shyla suffered from severe neglect as a puppy and has her own challenging and neurotic relationship with food. At the park, I met a lovely young woman by the name of Haley. She had recently moved back to Austin after spending a few years in New York pursuing a career in advertising. She was tall, friendly, beautiful, curvy, and dressed with discernibly more sophistication than the average casual Austinite. We easily struck up a conversation.

She asked me what I "did", and I explained I was writing a book to help people transform their relationship to food. She smiled and said, "Well, I need to read that!"

She began to tell me about her developing interest in food and nutrition. She had dipped her toe in the water, but felt she had a big dive ahead of her. Haley described her mother's metamorphosis after recently changing her diet, which eliminated the need for many of the medications she had been taking for decades.

7 Jena Hilliard, "Study Reveals Gen Z as the Loneliest Generation in America," Addiction Center. accessed May 22, 2021, https://www.addictioncenter.com/news/2019/08/gen-z-loneliest-generation/

I could tell it was a charged topic for her – both refreshing and nerve-racking to share. I asked her what she felt she needed. She answered, somewhat shyly, "It's really my *relationship* with food that needs help."

The serendipity of the conversation was precious, as I had just taken a break from my writing. I'd hit a point in the creative process where my insecurities and uncertainties were mounting an internal uprising. *What if my book flops? Am I really a good enough writer to do this? Is this really what people need? Is it going to help anyone?*

It felt as if the universe plopped us down together on this muddy grassy plot of earth as a mirror of encouragement for one another.

As I inquired deeper about her relationship dynamics with food, I could see tears glistening down her cheeks from my socially distanced position.

She detailed the lineage of eating disorders among the women in her family, spoken and unspoken. She explored the micro-traumas and messages that had informed her own eating habits. She reminisced about the fast food she grew up eating, and the anger she felt at her mother for feeding her such crap. Then she expressed the guilt she felt about harboring resentment toward her mother, who she knew was doing the best she *could* at the time.

Haley shared her odd cravings and aversions of certain foods. For her, texture is imperative. Anything unctuous or slimy is completely repulsive to her. Food must have a perfect balance of dry, crunch, and pungency for her to eat it. She also recognized how she uses food both as reward and punishment for herself. She'd been told that her habits resemble ARFID, avoidant-restrictive food intake disorder, but wasn't sure she wanted to go down the path of labelling herself with an eating disorder.

Virtually everything she had been told about food as a young person now seemed like a mistruth. She recognized that much of the "good advice" that she received growing up was actually nutritional propaganda and emotional fear mongering.

After an hour together, she said something that hit me right in the heart. Another tear dropped down her rosy cheek as she sighed, "I love cooking, I just don't like cooking *alone*."

She reflected back to the satisfaction she felt while living with her roommate in New York. They often cooked, ate, and laughed together. Haley's eating habits were much healthier then. She talked wistfully about her brother, whose family created healthy and fulfilling food habits that strike a balance between sustenance and desire. She recognized how her relationship with food reflected the lack of community in her everyday life.

Haley is certainly not alone in her loneliness. It's no wonder that so many people opt to eat out rather than cook these days.

Haley and I had both walked to the park empty handed – no cell phones, business cards, pen, or paper. We shared our names before we parted ways, and I verbally gave her my email. I felt like giving her a giant hug, but didn't out of respect for COVID-19 social distancing. Instead, I told her I would love to cook with her sometime. She thanked me for what she called an "impromptu therapy session," and we gestured to see each other again at the dog park.

Healing the Wounds of Lost Connection

I am a big believer in the power of community. I also know the challenges of it. I love the idea of the big happy family, the boisterous cheer of the Tuscan table, and the camaraderie of communities coming together to solve global problems. I also know the reality of abusive power dynamics, economic disparity, and contradictory values that lead to blame and separation. Family and harmonious community seem to be more of a rarity than a commonality today.

We all know what it feels like to be physically alone, as well as the disquieting sense of feeling alone amidst a crowd of people. Aloneness and loneliness are two starkly different experiences. We are living in a time with an abundance of opportunity for connection, and yet, we are the loneliest we have ever been. The experience of connection has an enormous effect on our bodies and brains.

For example, addiction appears to be intimately linked to our experience of loneliness and connection. In 2018, the researchers at NIDA Intramural Research Program gave rats the option of pressing one lever for a drug infusion or a different lever to open a door and interact with a social peer. The rats opted to open the door more than 90 percent of the time – even when they had previously self-administered methamphetamine for many days and exhibited behaviors that correspond to human addictive behaviors![8] The study showed that social interactions can have a profound effect on drug use, relapse, and the brain's response to drug-associated cues. Rats and humans have very similar brains, and similar research has shown the irrefutable connection between addiction and the lack of fulfilling social connection in humans.

Food has been shown to elicit similar neurological responses as addictive drugs such as cocaine. Those who crave food uncontrollably and eat more than they'd planned appear to anticipate food in much the same way that drug addicts anticipate a fix. Similarly, if you look at a PET scan of the brain on sugar, it looks almost indistinguishable to the

---

8 Marco Venniro, Marco Zhang, Daniele Caprioli, Jennifer K. Hoots, Sam A. Golden, Conor Heins, Marisela Morales, David H. Epstein, and Yavin Shaham, "Volitional Social Interaction Prevents Drug Addiction in Rat Models," *Nature Neuroscience* 21, no. 11 (October 2018): 1520-1529.

image of a brain on cocaine. Sugar follows the same neurocircuitry as smoking, alcohol and drugs.[9]

Our food habits take on the personality of our feelings of connection and community. Humans are a social species, and food is something social species share. Sharing food, warmth, and ideas is a major part of the way we survive and thrive. Healthy food habits plummet in environments that feel isolating and threatening, be it physically or emotionally. They flourish in environments that feel safe and connected.

While unhealthy food habits can be a symptom of distress and loneliness, food can also serve as a vehicle to repair the wounds of lost connection. Through food, we have an opportunity to connect and serve every day.

~

After two full days of travel and a bumpy, four-hour taxi ride from the Mumbai airport, we arrived at our temporary residence at about 10:00 pm. Victor, my long-time partner in Ayurveda, and I were travelling to Pune, India to study with a beloved mentor of ours. We were gratefully renting a room at a traditional Indian Music School called Parivar, where our mentor had suggested we take residence.

---

9 Pamela McKay, Patrick Fielding, Eve Gallop-Evans, Georgina W. Hall, Jonathan Lambert, Mike Leach, Teresa Marafioti, Christopher McNamara, and British Committee for Standards in Haematology, "Guidelines for the investigation and management of nodular lymphocyte predominant Hodgkin lymphoma," *British Journal of Haematology* 172, no. 1 (2016): 32-43.

When we arrived, our host, Swapna, graciously offered to feed us. Tossing out our typical rules of no food after sundown, we accepted her offer. We were extremely hungry and hadn't enjoyed a real meal in a couple of days.

She brought us each a warm bowl of rice and daal – Indian lentil stew – seasoned to perfection. We ate and talked for at least an hour. We had come to a truly wonderful place.

As we neared the end of our conversation, ready to unpack and get to bed, she remarked how we were unlike most Americans who passed through. Swapna generally did not like hosting people from our country because they often felt cold and ungrateful. Many just expected to be served as though they were at a restaurant. She felt that we were truly interested in learning about India – its food, its people, and its traditions.

The act of receiving her offering, though it didn't fit our "rules", opened the door to a connection that we otherwise would have missed. The connection turned out to be one I will cherish for all my life.

The people at Parivar quickly became family to us. We met each day and enjoyed at least two meals together in between our Ayurvedic work and studies.

A prominent musician and educator herself, Swapna took in young musicians who struggled financially, offering them a place to live and home-cooked meals as they focused on honing their craft. She cooked fresh meals for them every day. She described it as part of her *seva* – her act of service. She knew the experience of sacrificing security to pursue talent and passion, and she thought everyone deserved healthy, warm food as they worked toward their dreams.

Her meals were incredible. They were simple but layered with depthful subtleties. I felt deeply nourished after every meal – not just in my belly, but in every part of me.

Swapna created a life in which she never cooked just for herself. It brought her joy. She did not serve others at the expense of herself. She was healthy and successful. Every day she fed herself with one hand and her community with the other.

On our way home from India, we stopped through Heathrow Airport in London. I remember the feeling of emptiness I felt when seeking a plastic-wrapped meal from the cold, mechanical kiosks. Everyone looked hurried and uninterested in one another. While my pre-packaged veggie wrap fed me nutritionally, it was missing the nourishing essence – the heart, the soul, and the communion – of where we had just been. My airport meal felt like a coloring sheet with outlines that were never colored in.

I missed the warmth – the color – I had fallen in love with. I became aware of the parts of my life that shared in that magical quality of *seva* I had experienced in India, and the parts that did not.

At the time, I lived in a yoga community in Northern California. For about a decade, we had set out to live more collectively, sustainably and consciously. We built a commercial kitchen that was attached to our Ayurvedic clinic where we cooked for each other, a few clients, and held an occasional cooking class.

A few months after returning home, we decided to ramp up the kitchen and offer Ayurvedic-inspired meals and vegan baked goods to our local community. A few months after that, we transitioned the kitchen to a nonprofit and offered all of our meals by donation. The kitchen got busier, served more people, got more press, and brought in more revenue.

The transformation of the kitchen mirrored a transformation in me for which I am deeply grateful. Spending part of my time each day feeding food to my community food I believed in kindled a fire of tremendous joy in me, a joy lit by the spark of inspiration from Swapna.

~

Not everyone has the desire or ability to serve food to a community of people every day. Fortunately, there are countless avenues of *offering*, born from the authentic desire to connect and share resources with one another. We have this opportunity every day, even in the most mundane activities.

Athena, a pediatric occupational therapist, recently shared with me how much she enjoyed mealtimes with her ten-month-old baby. *That's an astonishing feat*, I thought. So many parents have an absolute enmity for mealtime. Feeding time with children is often an anxiety riddled battleground for control and a disastrous mess, where more food ends up on the other side of the room than inside the child's mouth. Amidst a busy lifestyle, feelings of resentment and obligation quickly attach themselves to the chaos of breakfast, lunch, and dinner.

Athena loves watching her son, Andreas, discover and rediscover food. She never forces him to eat anything. She always offers two or three healthy options for him to play with, explore, and taste. Some days, he just loves sweet potatoes, and other days, he wants nothing to do with them. Then, a few days later he enthusiastically rediscovers them like a pirate discovering a chest of gems for the first time.

I whole-heartedly disagree with the common phrase "don't play with your food!" Play is how we connect most authentically to the world.

By observing the way Andreas responds to food offerings, she learns about him. She learns what he likes about the textures, temperatures, shapes, and combinations of food, and how they relate to his mood, biorhythms, and development. She influences his food choices by what she chooses to offer him, but allows him to accept or reject what goes in his body.

This helps Andreas learn to trust his own instincts and trust her as a caregiver. Plus, by allowing herself to *enjoy* the often-dreaded process of mealtime, she turns an arduous task into a pleasurable joy.

We all have this ability to enchant the mundane through the act of offering. Here are some ideas:

- Forego the typical "slap it in down in front of them" style. Offer a meal to a loved one in a way that is truly present and sprinkled with special touches. Practice this regularly.
- Invite someone over for a home cooked meal and for connection once a week.
- Volunteer to serve underprivileged people in your community.
- Start a composting system and transform food waste into food for soil and insects.
- Grow a garden and share your abundance with your community.
- Contribute in some way, physically or financially, to the billions of hungry people in the world.
- Accept the offering of another when it is offered to you.
- Connect with your local farmers and gardeners. Buy as much of your food from them as possible.
- Next time you eat alone, slow down. Connect with your food, your environment, and yourself. Notice the taste, the texture and the subtleties that you would miss by eating quickly with your mind on something else.

All of these can be done either as an act of obligation or devotion. Your intention and attitude are the essential ingredients. Experience by experience, we can transform our relationship with food and community by engaging with food as an offering.

How do you currently experience food as an offering in your life?

How do you experience your sense of community? Who would you like to connect to more? How?

What can you create as an offering today? How about something you can look forward to repeating regularly—daily, weekly, monthly?

Radical Self-Care

There are a thousand ways to kneel and touch the ground.

– Rumi

In many cultures around the world, people pray or chant ceremoniously before eating. This practice is both an act of gratitude for the sustenance, and a ritual to honor the element of fire. In Ayurveda, the word *agni* refers to one's *digestive fire.* It corresponds to the action of metabolism - the enzymes, microbiota, and myriad of functions involved in the digestion of food.

Food gets broken down and transformed into energy. The food you eat becomes the tissues in your body. Your bones, your hair, your eyes, your skin… all are created from the food you eat. It's amazing to think that part of that carrot you ate for dinner is going to become part of your eyes, isn't it? When we eat, we offer the food we consume to the quality of fire within us, trusting it to transform our meal into what our body needs.

Every time we eat we make an offering to ourselves. We choose how to give and receive this offering with the resources we have available. Will our offering be an elixir or a toxin? Will we nurture or neglect ourselves? Will we honor our inner fire and stop eating when we're no longer hungry? Will we choose to eat in safe, loving company, even if that's just ourselves? Every aspect of eating reflects the way we care, or do not care, for ourselves.

Self-care often elicits feelings of guilt or selfishness. "We could be spending our time caring for another, or making money!" nags the inner voice.

Caretaker burnout, physician burnout, adrenal fatigue syndrome, occupational sudden mortality, martyrdom – these are all symptoms of giving more energy than you are taking in. There are many expressions of this – be it physical, mental, or emotional.

Overindulgence and greed are the other end of the spectrum. Consuming more than you need leads to accumulation and toxicity. Taking more than you give eventually leads to resentful and unfulfilling relationships. Both sides are patterns that express a neglect in self-care.

Prioritizing the need for self-care in our culture is an act of rebellion. It's often relegated to a luxury reserved for the rich and privileged. I can tell you with certainty: it's not selfish, it's essential.

Proper food, adequate rest, emotional and spiritual connection, alone time, physical touch, movement, sunlight, acts of purification, creative play, and a sense of purpose are all avenues of self-care we need to live fulfilling and healthful lives. Your diet includes all of these things. It is everything you take in – food, liquid, air, and perceptions.

Self-care actually extends far beyond ourselves. As parents, children learn not from what we say, but what we *do*. Children embody beliefs about food by witnessing the way their caretakers *feel* about eating. The same is true for teachers and leaders. We pass down habits and mindsets, which become the threads of future generations.

Every time you sit down to eat is an opportunity for self-care. Your vote with your fork has a ripple effect. Whether you realize it or not, your actions impress upon your friends, family, community, coworkers, and even your chance encounters. The priority you give your body, mind, and soul is contagious.

Purification

Just like a tree sheds its leaves every Fall, we too, must regularly shed. Purification is itself an offering. What you give away transforms into something that feeds another. The first law of thermodynamics is that energy cannot be created or destroyed, it can only be transferred or transformed from one form to another.

When I look back at my eating disorder, labelled as *bulimia*, it's no coincidence that my chosen method of expurgation was vomiting. I was not just purging the food I had binged on. I was also trying to expel the words, concepts, punishments, and traumas I had taken in. My body and mind were rejecting what I had consumed. When I stopped feeling the need to stuff things in, I stopped having the urge to unnaturally purge them out.

Life, however, is never void of the need to purify. Stress, tough lessons, and toxins are part of life, all of which need to be processed and eliminated efficiently. We must regularly remove waste from our body and life. Our body does this naturally through many channels of purification—the bowels, sweat, urine, menstruation, and vomiting to name a few. What is taken in and either rejected, processed, or no longer needed is excreted.

We eliminate mentally and emotionally through rest, tears, and verbal processing. It's not a coincidence that we use the phrase "word vomiting." Interestingly, vomiting in both forms is another action tied directly to the mouth.

Purification is the act of sifting through what's no longer relevant and allowing matter or energy to flow out in order to make space for new life.

Food can be both nourishing and purifying. People use juicing, fasting, ketosis and a variety of other approaches to food-based purification. In Ayurveda, we craft personalized food plans that emphasize building the *agni*, the strength of the digestion, and simplifying the diet to allow the body to purify itself naturally again. If someone needs extra support for purification, we use a method called *Panchakarma* to loosen and purify deep-seated toxins. Diet plays a fundamental role once again. As a client's body changes, the diet recommendations do, too.

A healthy diet strikes a balance between nourishment and assisting the body's natural purification processes. Ideally, our own metabolic process should serve as our natural detoxification machine.

Purification isn't just an occasional cleanse. Removing that which no longer serves us is a daily practice. Drinking adequate water, eating plenty of vegetables, lubricating the system with healthy fats and oils, and calling upon specific properties of medicinal herbs and spices can support this balance. We must also purify mentally and emotionally. Meditation, nature walks, tai chi, yoga, massage, art, and devotional practices help us to purify the mind.

Here are some questions to consider. Are you:

- Struggling to lose weight, even though you are eating healthy portions?

- Having a hard time going to the bathroom regularly?
- Developing congestion, such as excess mucus?
- Regularly feeling heavy or lethargic?
- Experiencing skin breakouts like acne, rashes, or eczema?
- Feeling like your mind or information load is "stuffed too full"?

These are all signs that you are in need of purification.

In addition to addressing the physical symptoms with a qualified practitioner, take a look at the way you may be unconsciously *holding on* to things that are no longer serving you.

Is it time to let go of a relationship from the past?

A fear of money?

Is it time to change the way you use social media?

Would it benefit you to practice gratitude in place of worry?

Can you take responsibility for the choices you've made while recognizing that you cannot control the outcome of them?

If you have anxiety around food, or your body-image, take a look at the *belief systems* that you are holding on to that no longer serve you. Such as:

Are you holding onto an idealized image of yourself?

Are you trying to uphold someone else's expectations of you?

Are you perceiving threats that are no longer real?

Is it time to truly accept yourself as good enough and capable?

Relaxation techniques that focus on our natural mechanisms of release can support the process of letting go of the old and making space for the new, physically and emotionally. Below, I outline a simple exercise to relax the *jaw, rectum* and *diaphragm*. Releasing these three regions goes a long way. I consider them to be the *three gateways of freedom*. In yoga, they correspond to the three main *bandas* or "locks". Yogi's learn to consciously tighten and relax them, in order to move energy through their channels. With proper training and practice, bandas can be used to direct the Kundalini energy up the main and central channel of the body, called the *sushumna*, to the higher centers. When these higher centers are activated, it's possible to experience *moksha* - liberation or enlightenment.

To start, we are simply going to focus on the relaxation of these three gateways. They each act as switches for the parasympathetic-sympathetic response. In a state of relaxation, they encourage the *rest and digest* response, and allow waste to flow smoothly out of our bodies and mind.

The Three Gateways of Freedom

Relaxation Exercise

1. Lay down or sit comfortably and close your eyes. Rotate your shoulders back and down, and gently lift the sternum (the center and base of the chest). Allow the chest to open.

2. Relax your jaw. Let it soften and drop down. You can let your mouth open slightly if that feels natural. Allow your tongue to rest on the upper palate of the mouth.

3. With your eyes closed, focus your vision between your eyebrows. Allow your eyes to sink back into your head and "smile" with the back side of your eyes. Notice how this affects your jaw and cheeks.

4. Breathe into your belly, then exhale. On the exhale, contract your rectum and sex organs like you are stopping yourself from going to the bathroom. This is called *mulabhanda*, or "root lock" in yoga. Now release it and inhale. Really emphasize the relaxation of the anal sphincter. Do this three times. Relax a little deeper each time you release.

5. Keeping the rectum consciously relaxed, deepen and elongate your breath. First, fill the abdomen, then the chest with breath. Then let them both release together. Really allow your abdomen to extend outwards on the inhale, like a balloon that inflates your belly. Slow down your breath rhythm. Breathe as slow and elongated as possible, like you're breathing in slow motion.

Now just lay or sit totally relaxed in this state for 3 minutes or more. Repeat daily. If you have a regular meditation practice, you can integrate these practices into it to deepen your relaxation.

*You can find a guided recording of this exercise on my website - www.livewiseheal.com

When we are peaceful and calm, we can take time to look deeply into ourselves and into the situation we are in. When our mind and body are calm, we can see the situation more clearly. Our view is not obscured or distorted.

– Thich Nhat Hanh, "How to See"

When we receive nourishment and purify waste effectively, we create health and vitality. Like a city whose traffic flows smoothly, our energy flows unimpeded through our channels. We can give and receive circularly, without attachment or neglect. We can look outside of ourselves with as much compassion and clarity as we give ourselves.

Your FoodPrint

Have you ever thought about the lifecycle of the meal you are eating? What was the journey it embarked on to arrive on your plate? What elements were necessary to grow and produce it - the rain, the soil, the sunlight? Who were all of the people, companies and machines involved in the cultivation and distribution of it? How about the farmers, the producers, the drivers, and the grocers that contributed their energy to it? What distance was it transported to get to you?

Next time you eat, take a moment to consider all that has gone into what you are about to ingest. See if you can imagine the energy and offerings that have unfolded for it to be there with you.

You may begin to recognize the interconnectedness of the elements, people, and processes that contributed to bringing your food to you.

When you offer food to your body with this mindfulness, you may notice a natural sense of gratitude and reverence wash over you. You may notice a different feeling when you eat it. You may even notice that you naturally begin to desire different food.

~

Your *foodprint* is how your relationship to food affects both you and the rest of the world.

You may or may not be aware of how your food habits affect the world's resources, or how the dietary habits of the developed world intensely affect the rest of the globe. The mass production of dairy, meat, corn, soy and palm oil has a massive effect on the environment, on people living in third-world countries, and on indigenous communities around the world. [10]

Our habits of consumption have enormous implications beyond just our culinary preferences. Our industrialized packaging materials, namely Styrofoam and plastic, are now found in the deepest parts of our oceans. Every time you buy something wrapped in plastic, that packaging ends up somewhere that you likely don't see, yet. It will likely end up stuck in the belly of an aquatic animal, in part of the Great Pacific Garbage Patch, or as part of an unfathomably large trash landfill that is most likely exported to other countries.[11] The Great Pacific Garbage Patch is a trash gyre in the Pacific Ocean estimated to be about 1.6 million square kilometers and has been increasing 10-fold each decade since 1945.

Plastic, while possessing many impressive qualities, does not biodegrade. Instead, it breaks down into smaller and smaller pieces called microplastics. Microplastics are present in virtually all corners of the Earth and infiltrate the air we breathe, the food we eat, and the water we drink in truly alarming amounts. A recent study by the World Wildlife Fund (WWF) found that people could be consuming up to a credit card worth of plastic microparticles every week. That's about a dinner-plate worth of plastic every year.[12] Now that's a part of your daily "diet" you don't usually consider when you're counting your calories!

---

10 Erin Skoczylas, "Foodprint: How Our Diet Affects the Carbon Footprint," accessed January 16, 2021.

11 Livia Albeck-Rip, "The 'Great Pacific Garbage Patch' is ballooning, 87,000 tons of plastic and counting," *The New York Times,* March 22, 2018, https://www.nytimes.com/2018/03/22/climate/great-pacific-garbage-patch.html

12 Reuters, "A Plateful of Plastic," accessed 20 May, 2021, https://graphics.reuters.com/ENVIRONMENT-PLASTIC/0100B4TF2MQ/index.html

The chemicals found in plastics have been linked to a variety of health problems including reproductive abnormalities, lowered sperm count, obesity, and developmental delays in children. [13]

To make matters worse, plastics are made from petrochemicals, a refined derivative of petroleum. Petrochemicals are used to make materials for electronics, furniture, shoes, adhesive, medical supplies, sports goods, packaging, detergents, paints, paper, textiles, inks, construction, and pharmaceuticals[14]. They are rapidly becoming the largest driver of global oil consumption. As renewable energy sources like solar, wind and hydro-electric become more cost-effective than oil and gas, investment in plastic by oil and gas companies is ramping up.[15] Plastics are set to account for more than a third of the growth in oil demand by 2030, and nearly half by 2050. This is ahead of trucks, aviation and shipping.[16] Seventy-five percent of petrochemical production is for the manufacturing of more plastic.

The majority of plastic manufacturing plants are located in low-income communities. These communities face radically inequitable health effects from the offgasses of large manufacturing plants. In addition, manufacturing facilities in communities of color have

---

13 The Washington Post, "You're Literally Eating Microplastics. How You Can Cut Down Exposure to Them," accessed March 31, 2021, https://www.washingtonpost.com/health/youre-literally-eating-microplastics-how-you-can-cut-down-exposure-to-them/2019/10/04/22ebdfb6-e17a-11e9-8dc8-498eabc129a0_story.html

14 Nicola A. Hanania, Sidney Braman, Sandra G. Adams, Ruth Adewuya, Arzu Ari, JoAnn Brooks, Donald A. Mahler, Jill A. Ohar, Jay Peters, and Shahin Sanjar, "The Role of Inhalation Delivery Devices in COPD: Perspectives of Patients and Health Care Providers," *Chronic Obstructive Pulmonary Diseases: Journal of the COPD Foundation* 5, no. 2 (April 2018): 111.

15 Beth E. Gardiner, "The Plastics Pipeline: A Surge of New Production is on the Way," accessed September 1, 2021, https://e360.yale.edu/features/the-plastics-pipeline-a-surge-of-new-production-is-on-the-way

16 International Energy Agency, "Petrochemicals Set to be the Largest Driver of World Oil Demand, Latest IEA Analysis Finds," accessed January 16, 2021, https://www.iea.org/news/petrochemicals-set-to-be-the-largest-driver-of-world-oil-demand-latest-iea-analysis-finds

more than twice the rate of toxic release incidents than facilities in predominantly white communities.[17]

Next time you go to the grocery store, take a look at the amount of plastic in your cart. Recognize the consequences of our industrial habits, and the very real conundrum we find ourselves in.

Plastics and manufacturing are unfortunately not the only contributing industry to our environmental crisis. Meat production and industrial agricultural practices are leaders in this dystopian race. These two industries add up to more CO2 emissions than transportation and power generation. Detailed estimates tie 51 percent of CO2 emissions worldwide to meat and dairy production and distribution.[18]

Aside from the processing and transportation of meat and animal products, livestock requires vast swathes of land for grazing. It is projected that over 150 acres of land is lost in the Amazon every minute. That is more than one football field every second of every day. In the Amazon basin, up to 70 percent of this deforestation is attributed to cattle production.[19]

Scientists say deforestation is nearing a point of no return. What's left of the rainforest could become savannah within 50 years. The Amazon, considered the lungs of the world, is tied delicately to the climate. The respiration and the vitality of the entire planet, including you and me, depends on it.[20]

---

17 Center for Effective Government, *Living in the Shadow of Danger* (Michigan: W.K. Kellogg Foundation, 2016).

18 "Key Facts and Findings," Food and Agriculture Organization of the United Nations, accessed June 29, http://www.fao.org/news/story/en/item/197623/icode/

19 Esther Perel, *Mating in Captivity: Reconciling the Erotic and the Domestic* (New York: HarperCollins, 2006).

20 "Climate Change in the Amazon," World Wildlife Fund, accessed March 21, 2021, https://wwf.panda.org/discover/knowledge_hub/where_we_work/amazon/amazon_threats/climate_change_amazon/?

In addition to ecological collapse, the Amazon faces a humanitarian crisis that is less talked about. Five centuries ago, there were an estimated 10 million native Indians living in the Amazonian rainforest. Today, there are less than 200,000. In Brazil alone, European colonists have destroyed more than 90 indigenous tribes since the 1900s.[21]

A similar trend is present today in the rainforests of Borneo, where the majority of the world's palm oil is derived. Palm oil is widely used in food products, detergents and cosmetics. Borneo is home to one of the oldest and largest rainforests in the world, a variety of endemic and endangered species, and a variety of indigenous tribes. The rapid and extensive destruction of the forest for palm oil production threatens them all. Fifty percent of the lowland rainforest is gone.[22] The genocide and habitat destruction occurring in Borneo, South America, and fertile land across the globe is unthinkable.

We haven't even begun talking about chemical fertilizers, antibiotics, radiation, genetic modification, and soil degradation that affects the food supply and fuels both humanitarian and ecological crises. We must become aware of the way our food habits and our food production impact our personal and collective well-being. We must take part in demanding and creating new models.

Reversing this crisis is a complex and enormous task that cannot be solved by replacing one unsustainable system with another. It requires a dramatic and widespread change in government legislation. It depends on businesses and corporations creating sustainable manufacturing practices and energy production. It challenges our economy to embrace the principles of ecological economics. It necessitates banks to direct

21 "About the Rainforest", Rain-Tree Publishers, accessed August 15, 2021, https://rain-tree.com/facts.htm

22 "About the Rainforest", Rain-Tree Publishers, accessed August 15, 2021, https://rain-tree.com/facts.htm

funding away from resource extraction and toward projects that focus on the regeneration of the environment and local communities. It beckons consumers like you and me to stand loud and consistent in our demand. It calls us to uphold our sustainable lifestyle practices. It also requires consumers to be willing not just to talk about better choices, but be willing to pay more for them as needed.

Living dominantly plant-based lifestyles, supporting regenerative agriculture practices, reducing consumption, and supporting local food production are all votes we can cast with our forks everyday.

I know the reality is depressing and complex. It's easy to feel powerless, like you cannot drink a cup of coffee or eat a meal without oppressing something or someone. This is what makes engaging with the truth of your *foodprint* so difficult. However, we can choose to relate to it with passion and honesty.

While it's frustrating to me that it is virtually impossible to leave the market without some sort of plastic in my cart, the urgency of this crisis inspires me to think differently. I am drawn to find new solutions and start conversations about the problem at hand. The depressing reality urges me to organize, educate, and be part of a solution. In turn, my relationship with food takes on meaning and purpose that extends far beyond just my own nourishment or desire.

Our relationship to food spans across so many facets of life – personal, cultural, and environmental. Just like with health, there is no one-size-fits-all solution – it is always contextual.

Remember, everything in nature is medicinal if used in a balanced way, and toxic if used in an imbalanced way.

I encourage you to educate yourself even when it feels easier to leave challenging topics behind the veil. Question the sources of your information, the funding behind the sources, and the motives behind the funding. Challenge yourself to build new habits that take yourself *and* the collective into consideration. Ask yourself – "What *foodprint* would I like to leave on myself and on the world?" Afterall, we are inextricably interconnected.

Start with what you care most about – be it your children, animals, your health, your local community, etc. Learn about the way your food habits impact its well-being. If your values don't line up with your actions, or if perhaps your cravings don't match the disposition of your heart, then get creative. Have some fun crafting solutions that make you feel whole.

Just like any other system of oppression that exists in the world, big change does not happen overnight. Stay with it. Know that what feeds your heart also feeds the heart of the world.

"Happiness is when what you think, what you say,

and what you do are in harmony."

– Mahatma Gandhi

Your Life's Offering

Upon our arrival to the other side of the world, the very first thing they did was feed us. The Tongan people seemed eager to teach us about their native food traditions. They offered us as much as we could possibly consume of their cuisine. They even showed us how to open a coconut in midair with a machete.

The Kingdom of Tonga is an island monarchy in the South Pacific. Most in the West know of it only by its reputation for creating sought-after football and rugby players. Tongans are historically some of the largest and strongest people on the planet. They are often recruited for professional athletics, and they have lineages of queens that were more than seven feet tall.[23]

Roosters and pigs meandered free on the land where we stayed, a stark contrast to the honking cars and hustling people back home. I will never forget the "cock-a-doodle-doos" just inches from my bedside wall in the wee hours of the morning. Talk about an effective alarm clock! The sound reminded me how much of nature existed only as theory from children's books and nursery rhymes in my life.

To bathe, we collected cold, slow-dripping water in buckets from the shower faucet. This chilling reality made me starkly aware of both my privileged comforts and our haphazardly wasteful habits.

A bell rang at the same time each day. Everyone on the island stopped whatever they were doing and stood in silence for one minute before returning to their daily tasks. That mere minute of silence was like pressing the reset button on an electronic device. It seemed to systemically refresh everyone's circuits. Peace, beauty, and reverence naturally washed through my channels. This daily practice permanently made its mark on me.

We were taken into jungles and sweeping coastal plains. We witnessed bands of wild horses, and prehistoric plants and animal species. We interacted with the local people and learned about the religious colonization and economic westernization the nation faced. I fell in love with the ecological and cultural richness all around me.

I came to Tonga with four other amazing women as part of a project to teach dance and therapeutic movement to young adults who had been victims of sexual or physical assault. Our offering

23 "Tonga," wikipedia, accessed March 2, 2021, https://en.wikipedia.org/wiki/Tonga

was surprisingly well received, and inspired all five of us to continue exploring the therapeutic benefits of movement in our various careers in healthcare. In retrospect, we certainly gained as much from the people and land of Tonga as we offered to them.

Coming back to the U.S., I experienced a bad case of reverse culture shock. The dissonance I felt initiated a turning point that informed the choices and life I envisioned for myself thereafter. In Tonga, I realized there were many aspects of my own culture that I had passively accepted as simply "the way things are." My travels opened my eyes to the wisdom of indigenous people, the wealth of nature, and the countless ways we can live and serve. It showed me that funding exists for work that is meaningful to me. My time there curated a new perspective of culture, showing me that traditions are created through a collective acceptance of shared values. Instead of passively complying, I can choose which values I want to live by.

My relationship with food really shifted alongside this big pivot in my life's focus. I intentionally stopped trying to "fit in" to the blueprint of cultural standards I thought I needed to adhere to. I began to follow the sparks of my own interests, gifts, and curiosities, and I saw inequities and imbalances that I wanted to be part of restoring. My life's work, my *offering*, began to unfold.

I personally notice a direct correlation between my eating habits and my alignment to my *truth*. When there is incongruity between my actions and my values, my eating habits start to wobble. When I am centered in how I intend to serve, food becomes a tool to sustain that mission and a pleasure to enjoy along the way.

Food becomes an ally, rather than an antagonist, as we (food and I) both share a common purpose of *offering* our beneficence to those who accept it.

People often say to me: "I don't know what my *purpose* is." From my perspective, a strong sense of purpose is paramount for health and happiness. The lack thereof is a major theme I observe among people suffering with chronic illness.

Purpose comes in many forms. It may manifest as a lifelong commitment to fulfill a focused mission or project. It may be the cultivation of a specialized skill combined with an attitude of service that takes on many expressions. Purpose goes beyond a striving for money or status. It's not necessarily grand and won't guarantee riches or fame. It's not idealistic or ungrounded. Your purpose gets you up in the morning. It's what you live for.

Your purpose stems from a quality of *being*, a state of genuinity and a generosity that infuses everything you do. It weaves together your unique gifts and interests and imbues you with passion to serve the world around you. The deeper you know yourself, the more potency you have to bring your personal mission to life.

While uncovering purpose is certainly not a linear thought process to be tackled overnight, the intersection of these four questions can help guide you in the unfolding of your life's offering.

What do you love?

What gifts do you have?

What do you think the world around you needs most?

How can you make money bringing these to form?

Whether you are a young person, middle-aged, or a wizened elder – It is never too late to offer your gifts and kindness as food to the world around you. It may even take a new form today than it did earlier in your life.

Our life's offering is an act of creation, whether we enjoy the fruits of our labor or not. Similar to a gardener who plants trees but may never live to see them fully grown, we plant our own seeds of energy and inspiration simply because our soul is called to do so. The full impact of our offering is up to forces beyond our control. The fulfillment we gain lies in the journey of bringing it forward. Collectively, we have the potential to grow a forest that provides shade for generations to come.

~

When we stand for the well-being of all, not just in self-interest, our biggest challenges and inherent gifts alchemize into *offerings*. Rooted in loving kindness, offerings come in infinite forms – interpersonal communication, writing, art, activism, and business. An empowered voice combined with an empowered heart is a powerful combination that can be expressed through all of these mediums. Leadership, in the spirit of offering, is an act of servitude.

For much of history, we have seen empowered voices with *un*empowered hearts. Voices who have commanded movements to colonize, kill, suppress, and silence whole sectors of the human race – as well as animals, the environment, and ocean life. We have experienced time and time again the destructive use of power.

It is easy to associate power with greed, thinking power is inherently used destructively. We need a new definition of power, one that heeds the voices of inclusivity, balance, and peace.

Underneath bigotry, oppression, and violence lives a wounded heart. Wounded people wound people. This does not excuse acts of violence, but it does beckon for a compassionate reassessment of the causation that builds the foundation for personal and collective cycles of violence. As we offer compassion to our own wounds, we craft ourselves into a vessel for generosity. We can then offer the same opportunity to others – even those who have committed the most seemingly unforgivable crimes.

At its center, the profession of healing is the fulfillment of our wish to serve, to give – and to be restored. Outwardly, we direct our efforts toward restoring others, but somewhere maybe we know that there really is no other.

- Saki Santorelli,
Heal Thyself: Lessons on Mindfulness in Medicine

Setting Sail

As we undergo a depthful exploration into our relationship with food, we also delve into the caverns within ourselves. Each part of the terrain is valuable and insightful, if we let it be.

This dance of *sustenance*, *pleasure* and *offering* is both primal and sacred. Your life will continue to present you the opportunity to waltz your way through the ebbs and flows with each of them. You are not required to know the steps. You are simply called to accept the invitation to dance.

Food offers us the chance to connect with our bodies, our minds, our communities, and our Earth every day. It invites us to love ourselves and the world around us with each meal. It summons us to sustain the spark that lives within us.

In a balanced relationship, we don't take more than we need. We don't give more than we have. We play. We learn. We invite nourishment physically, mentally, and spiritually.

Your diet is not just a map of a food pyramid. It is as unique as you are. It consists of everything you *take in*. You become everything you *digest*. Your wellness depends on how well you *release* what you no longer need.

As you go through the process of fine-tuning the food that truly nourishes you, remember to check back in with your breath. Keep that stress response harnessed in the passenger seat, rather than as the captain of your ship.

Remember that your unique body shape and size, as nature made it, is beautiful.

Remember that en*joy*ment is sacred, not sinful.

Remember the power you have to vote with your fork.

Remind yourself not to take anything too seriously. Radical honesty paired with an air of lightheartedness is a powerful catalyst for change. As Esther Perel puts it, remember to *acknowledge your flaws and still hold yourself in high regard.*

Food may have once taken on a variety of meanings and masks. It does not need to remain that way. Perhaps it is time to re-write the agreement you made many moons ago. You have the tools at your fingertips. You have the wisdom and the wherewithal. You deserve to create a loving and passionate relationship that feeds you on all levels – mind, body & soul.

I wish you the very best on this beautiful journey.

~

The following Workbook section includes an *Ayurvedic Body Constitution Assessment*, dietary and lifestyle recommendations for each *dosha* type, recommended staples for creating a healing kitchen, and a few key recipes. Keep an eye out for the Mind Body Food Recipe Book – coming soon!

Madison offers virtual and in-person consultations,
classes, and events worldwide.
@livewise_madisonmadden
www.livewiseheal.com

WORKBOOK:

CREATING A HEALING KITCHEN

If diet is wrong, medicine is of no use.
If diet is correct, medicine is of no need.

Ayurvedic Proverb

Ayurvedic Dosha Assessment

There is no one-size-fits-all when it comes to diet. Knowing your dominant constitution is an important step toward understanding which foods to emphasize and which to minimize. Your constitution refers to the unique bio-elemental balance that you were born with and which expresses your body-mind condition. It is assessed from physical traits, physiological tendencies, and psychological characteristics. In Ayurveda, your constitution is made up of a unique proportion of the three *doshas*. Doshas refer to the three fundamental bio-elemental forces that are termed – *vata, pitta*, and *kapha*. While there is much more depth and complexity to this topic than I will go into here, the three doshas break down as follows:

Kapha: Potential energy, cohesion, structure, anabolism (elements: water/earth)

Pitta: Thermal energy or bio-chemical energy, heat, metabolism (elements: fire/water)

Vata: Kinetic energy or movement, catabolism (elements: air/ ether)

Everyone has all three doshas within them. In fact, the three doshas are present in every cell of the human body. Their symbiosis forms a cornerstone of all life. Their proportion, and how they interact, is what we refer to as your constitution. Almost all of us have a dominant dosha, and often a subdominant dosha. Think of your constitution as the recipe that you are born with. The more you are able to align your diet and lifestyle to your unique constitution, the less likely you are to fall ill. The farther you stray from it, the more prone to illness you become. While many factors of life change and evolve over time, your constitution stays consistent.

Doshas are not just elements of the human body – they can be found all around us. If you start observing the rhythms of nature you will see the fundamental interplay of the doshas. Nature builds, transforms, and erodes in the cycle of kapha > pitta > vata in every micro and macrocosmic living system.

A tree, for instance, goes through its anabolic (building structure) stage in the Spring. It goes through its main stage of metabolism (transformation with heat) as it flowers and fruits in the Summer months. In the Fall, it begins its catabolic process of drying and shedding its fruit and leaves. It repeats this cycle for its lifespan. Daily biorhythms, the life cycle, the menstrual cycle, and the digestive process are all examples that also illustrate this elemental cycle.

I'll admit that I was reluctant to put a dosha assessment in this book. My attempt to make a complex concept digestible without oversimplifying is a delicate undertaking. I've witnessed self-assessment accidentally misguide more than a few well-intentioned health seekers. It is quite easy to mistake a characteristic of "imbalance" as a defining characteristic of your natural state. A busy electrician might self-identify as dominantly *pitta*, when his natural constitution is *kapha*. A new mother might mistakenly interpret that her nurturing and slower moving disposition since childbirth is *kapha*, when she is naturally more *vata*.

I've chosen to include the assessment anyway to offer a tool for you to begin applying the concepts we've discussed in a personalized way. I encourage you to review your findings with an Ayurvedic professional, who can help make important discernments that could be vital for your path of healing.

Below is your dosha assessment quiz. Underneath the quiz, you will find information about how the doshas are commonly expressed, as well as dietary recommendations for people with a dominance in each dosha. Ideally, an Ayurvedic professional would make recommendations specific to each person, but this will give you a sample platter of valuable insight to get you started.

Self-Assessment Quiz

For each line, mark the characteristic that most closely resembles you from three columns on the right. Choose characteristics that are closest to your lifelong experience over those that have only recently been present.

My physical body naturally has:	Thin build, small bones, small features	Medium build, defined muscle tone, sharp features	Thicker frame, rounded features, dense bones
When stressed, I tend towards:	Nervousness, fear	Anger, envy, jealousy	Sentimentality, sadness, attachment to the past
My appetite is:	Variable, sometimes strong sometimes gone	Strong, I get irritable when I'm not fed quickly	Mentally strong. I love eating but can get by with one good meal. I can feel heavy after eating
Weight, for me, is:	Hard to gain	Fairly easy to gain or lose, but stays relatively consistent	Hard to lose

I often crave:	Crunchy, munchy, dry foods	Salty, sour, spicy foods	Sweet, heavy, oily foods
I tend towards:	Gas, bloating, intestinal pain	Heartburn, acid reflux, burning sensations	Heaviness, lethargy, weight gain
My memory is:	Quick to learn, easy to forget	Sharp, average	Slower to learn, but remember forever
In communication, I tend to:	Talk quickly, sometimes nervous/shy	Be very direct, ok with confrontation	Speak softly, slowly, often the "peacemaker"
I love work that is:	Creative	Challenging	Routine
Routines are:	Hard to maintain	Well-organized even when they are shifting	Very habitual, without much effort
My skin tends towards:	Dryness	Redness, sensitivity, rashes	Softness, lustrous, moistness, pus
I feel thirsty:	Rarely, sometimes I forget to drink water	A lot	Moderate
I sweat:	In small amounts	Prolifically	I have to work for it

My bowel movements are:	Irregular, tend towards constipation	2+ times per day, tend towards looseness	1x per day, regular, large and well-formed
I often/sometimes:	Wake around 3-4 am	Wake up around 12-2 am	Have a hard time waking up in the morning
During the night, I often/sometimes experience:	Restlessness/ anxiety	Racing thoughts, to-do lists	Heavy sleep, lethargy
My body temperature tends to be:	Cold	Hot	Warm/clammy
I would describe one of my best attributes as:	Creativity, vision	Passionate, action-oriented	Nurturing, caring
TOTAL (add each column)	***Vata***	***Pitta***	***Kapha***

Which column has your highest score? Was one much higher than the rest? Was there a clear second place? It is possible to have a tridoshic constitution, in which all three are equally distributed, though this is rare.

Split your scores proportionally into percentages. Let's say my score looks like this:

Vata: 6

Pitta: 10

Kapha: 2

To get my percentages, I divide each score by 18 (the # of questions above).

Vata: 33%

Pitta: 56%

Kapha: 11%

In this example, my dominant constitution is *pitta*, and secondarily *vata*. I would then follow guidelines outlined for *pitta*, while also considering what keeps *vata* in balance. We often fall out of balance in the direction of our constitution, though it is possible to have a disease or imbalance in a dosha that is not your constitution. For instance, I could be a *pitta* with a *kapha* imbalance. I highly recommend you seek support from a clinical practitioner for these more complex pathologies. If you're not sure which of your tendencies are expressions of imbalance, and which are your innate constitution, this is also a good topic to discuss with a practitioner.

Below I outline simple diet and lifestyle recommendations for each dosha. These are general recommendations that do not account for personal variances. They are meant to act as a springboard, rather than a rule book. Recommendations for each dosha could fill an entire book.

Diet and Lifestyle Recommendations for Vata

Those with *vata* constitutions tend to be slender, sensitive, and possess extremely high creative vision. Elementally, vata is composed of air and ether. When balanced, *vata* types are full of joy and enthusiasm. They have keen intuition and have a tendency to act on impulse. When out of balance, they tend towards dryness, overexertion, depletion, anxiety, worry, insomnia and digestive issues like constipation, gas and bloating. Digestion tends to be irregular. They are usually sensitive to cold. Concentration can be difficult, and therefore they tend to have erratic habits. Eating and self-nurturing are usually irregular as well. While they may resist it, *vata* types secretly love and need to be nurtured. Structure and routine are very beneficial, though challenging to create. Slow, grounding, and rejuvenative practices such as yin yoga, nature walks, warm baths, oil massage, acupuncture, and tai chi are great. Vatas should emphasize warm food and drink. The vata dosha is involved in virtually all chronic and degenerative conditions, and increases naturally with age. For those with vata in their constitution, and for most people age 65-plus, these are beneficial guidelines to follow:

Qualities	Warm, moist, unctuous, moderately heavy, soothing, nourishing
Tastes	Prioritize sweet, sour and salty tastes. Avoid excess bitter, astringent and spicy tastes.

Grains & Legumes	Grains can be eaten in higher proportion. Prioritize organic whole grains like rice, oat, quinoa, millet, amaranth, buckwheat, and wheat. Minimize "dry" grain products like rice cakes, crackers and popcorn. Small legumes are best, such as split mung bean, lentil (red, green, brown, black), and adzuki beans. Other legumes and beans should be taken in smaller quantities and cooked with plenty of spices.
Dairy Products	Dairy products in moderate quantities can be balancing, especially ghee, milk and goat milk products. For vegans, emphasize nut milks, avocado, and coconut products.
Vegetables & Fruit	Squashes (zucchini, pumpkin, seasonal squashes), asparagus, beets, carrot, celery, cilantro, cucumber, daikon radish, green bean, okra, olive, cooked onion, parsnip, rutabaga, turnip, cooked spinach, cooked leafy greens, parsley, leek, cabbage, green chile. Grape, cherry, melon, peach, avocado, coconut, banana, orange, pineapple, plum, mango, papaya, apple, apricot, date, fig, lemon, lime, soaked raisin, rhubarb.
Nuts & Seeds	Flax, chia, pumpkin, sesame, poppy, sunflower seeds. Nuts in moderation, including: almond, walnut, Brazil nut, macadamia nut, coconut, hazelnut, peanut (this is actually a legume), pecan, pistachio, pine nut.

Spices	Cumin, coriander, fennel, cardamom, cinnamon, clove, allspice, basil, anise, star anise, black pepper (in moderation), curry leaf, dill, ajwain, garlic, ginger, marjoram, mint, mustard seed, nutmeg (moderation), oregano, paprika, parsley, long pepper, rosemary, thyme, turmeric, salt, hing, saffron, tarragon, vanilla.
Teas	Fennel, chamomile, ginger, licorice, lemon, fenugreek, lemongrass, marshmallow, peppermint, rosehip, raspberry, cardamom.
Avoid/Minimize	Cold, raw, rough, dry foods. Old food (leftovers), caffeine, fizzy drinks, junk food, cheese, junk food, processed sugar.
Lifestyle	Eat at regular times. Sit down and eat quietly, focusing on the taste and texture of your food. Chew thoroughly. Walk after each meal, at least 100 steps. Keep exercise gentle and regulated, and focus on balancing postures. Avoid excess windy, cold and dry environments. Drink two liters of water every day, emphasizing room temperature or warm water. Allocate time for expressing your creativity. Create time for rest, reflection, and nurturing. Maintain consistent routines.

Diet and Lifestyle Recommendations for Pitta

People with pitta-dominant constitutions usually run warm or hot, and have strong appetites and metabolism. They are typically orderly, focused, competitive, and athletic. They like to be in command. Balanced *pitta* types are passionate, assertive, and self-confident. They have natural leadership capabilities. When imbalanced, they can be pushy, demanding, impatient and angry. Elementally, pitta is composed of fire and water. Those with *pitta* constitutions (or imbalances) tend towards inflammatory conditions such as skin sensitivities and rashes, ulcers, heartburn, acid reflux, burning sensations, insomnia, vision/eye-problems, and arthritis. They also tend toward baldness or early graying, which is related to excess heat in the head region. Pitta-types often crave substances that fuel their fire, like coffee or spicy meals, which needs to be moderated to avoid burnout and inflammatory conditions. Cooling and calming practices are balancing for people with this constitution.

Qualities	Cooling, calming, luke-warm food/drink, need more protein than other constitutions.
Tastes	Sweet, bitter, astringent (minimize hot, sour, pungent, oily, fried, salty and fermented foods, as well as alcohol and coffee).
Grains & Legumes	Oats, rice, spelt, wheat, tapioca, amaranth, barley, couscous, coconut flour, mung beans, adzuki beans, black beans, black-eyed-peas, chick-peas, kidney beans, pinto beans, soybeans, split peas, tempeh, tofu, white beans, lima beans.

Dairy Products	Ghee, butter, soft cheeses, cow's milk, goat's milk, almond milk, rice milk, coconut milk, coconut yogurt.
Vegetables & Fruits	Cucumber, cabbage, sweet potato/yam, zucchini, leafy greens, pumpkin, artichoke, beets, bitter melon, bitter gourd, broccoli, Brussels sprouts, cauliflower, celery, cilantro, parsley, green beans, lettuce, okra, olives, parsnip, pea, sweet peppers, radish. Sweet fruits, such as - apple, avocado, sweet berries, sweet cherry, coconut, date, fig, grape, guava, lychee, mango, melons, papaya, pear, persimmon, plum, pomegranate, raisin.
Nuts & Seeds	Flax, pumpkin seeds, sunflower seeds, almonds (soaked and peeled), coconut.
Spices	Coriander, fennel, cilantro, fresh basil, cardamom, cinnamon, cumin, curry leaf, dill, ginger (in moderation), mint, parsley, saffron, wintergreen, turmeric.
Teas	Fennel, licorice, rose, tulsi, barley, borage, burdock, chamomile, chicory, comfrey, hibiscus, jasmine, dandelion, green tea, lavender, passion flower, brahmi, gotu kola, marshmallow, nettle, peppermint, raspberry, raspberry leaf, triphala, lemongrass.
Avoid/Minimize	Spicy foods, fried foods, excess oil, cheese, excess tomatoes, garlic, chili, sour fruits, feed, seafood, egg yolk.

Lifestyle	Approach everything with an attitude of moderation. Enjoy plenty of fresh air, nature, and fresh fruits and vegetables. Avoid overindulgence in sense organs. Practice daily meditation and quiet, contemplative practices. Keep body and head cool. Avoid situations of excess heat (steam, humidity, hot climates, etc.). Avoid a sedentary life.

Diet and Lifestyle Recommendations for Kapha

People with kapha-dominant constitutions usually have an easy-going, slow-paced and stable demeanor. They are generally affectionate, loving, and reliable. Physically, they are strong with a naturally heavier build and firm endurance. Elementally, kapha is built from water and earth. Balanced kapha-types have strong immune systems, strong long-term memory, and stable emotions. When imbalanced, they can be lethargic, apathetic, overly sentimental, and possessive. Kapha-dominant people tend to have sluggish digestion, and are prone to becoming overweight and heavily depressed. Physically, they are prone to conditions of excess such as: mucus/congestion, tumors, growths, high cholesterol, atherosclerosis, diabetes, edema, aching joints and heavy limbs. It is vital for people with kapha in their constitution to keep their diet light, eat only as much as they can digest each meal, and prioritize regular and strenuous physical activity.

Qualities	Warm, light, dry, slightly stimulating
Tastes	Pungent, bitter, astringent. Avoid excess sweet and salty tastes.

Grains & Legumes	Barley, corn, millet, buckwheat, rye, wheat bran, oats, wild rice, sprouted wheat, couscous, durham flour, and most legumes/beans including: adzuki, black beans, garbanzo, lentils, lima, mung, pinto, white beans, tofu.
Dairy Products	Minimize dairy products. Small amounts of goat's milk, goat cheese, and ghee are better options.
Vegetables & Fruits	Eggplant, beetroot and greens, leafy greens (cooked), cucumber, radish, green bean and pea, bitter melon, broccoli, cauliflower, Brussels sprouts, green chili, horseradish, kohlrabi, leeks, lettuce, arugula, sprouts, tomatoes, wheatgrass. Astringent and dry fruits including: apple, pomegranate, pear, fig, rhubarb, raisin, cranberry, cherry, prune, persimmon. Dried fruits in moderation are good choices.
Nuts & Seeds	Sunflower seeds, flax seeds, pumpkin seeds, chia, popcorn (avoid butter and salt), poppy seed. Nuts take in small quantities.
Spices	Liberal amounts of spices including: basil, ajwain, anise, bay leaf, black pepper, white pepper, caraway, cardamom, cayenne, clove, cinnamon, coriander, cumin, curry leaf, fill, fenugreek, methi, garlic, ginger, mace, marjoram, mustard seed, neem, nutmeg, oregano, paprika, rosemary, parsley, pippali, sage, savory, star anise, tarragon, hing, thyme, turmeric, mint.

Teas	Peppermint, fenugreek, ginger, cinnamon, black tea, green tea, white tea, tulsi, cardamom.
Avoid/Minimize	Excess salt and sweet tastes. All processed sugar. All fried foods. Excessive white flour, cheese, yogurt, banana, mango, watermelon, oil, beef, pork, seafood, rice, noodles, bread, iced drinks, desserts.
Lifestyle	Wake early (before sunrise). Avoid sleeping during the day. Exercise daily and break a sweat. Invite challenge, excitement & novelty. Keep warm and dry. Avoid excessively moist environments. Avoid a sedentary life.

Staples for a Healing Kitchen

Here are a few of my staples for outfitting a kitchen fit for delicious, compassionate, and digestible meals! I often cook multicultural meals, and I am vegetarian. I opt for organic and locally sourced whenever possible.

I encourage you to play and experiment with spices, flavors, and combinations. Food should not be a chore. Allow yourself to be creative, enjoy new flavors, and find ways to make the flavors you love healing for you! Everyone's healing kitchen will be unique,

This section has been largely inspired by my long-time mentor and kitchen partner, Joe.

A Wealth of Spices

Spices have been deemphasized in modern cooking. Many spice cabinets are decorated with just garlic, onion, salt, and pepper. However, herbs and spices have been a beloved and vital part of traditional cooking around the world for centuries. Many foods, such as legumes, have always been cooked with a generous number of spices to enhance their digestibility.

Each herb or spice has a unique profile of flavor, aroma, and medicinal qualities. Spices can be used in a variety of combinations in virtually every meal.

I've listed my top 20 spices in alphabetical order. I recommend prioritizing the spices that match your dosha assessment. You can learn much more about each of these spices in the book *Healing Spices* by Bharat B. Aggarwal, PhD.

I recommend buying these in bulk and storing them in glass containers for easy spooning. I encourage you to spice much more liberally than you think you should. *Play* with them!

Ajwain
Basil
Black Cumin Seeds
Black Peppercorn (Malabar)
Cardamom
Coriander
Clove
Cinnamon
Cumin
Fennel
Fenugreek and Methi (seed and leaf)
Ginger
Hing (Asafoetida)
Lemongrass
Mustard Seed
Oregano
Sage
Smokey Paprika
Thyme
Turmeric

**The Big 3: *Cumin, Coriander, Turmeric*

I like to keep a mixture of equal parts cumin, coriander and turmeric premade. This "big 3" mixture is my go-to digestive spice mix that can be added to virtually anything I cook to add a digestive and anti-inflammatory quality! I can layer on other spices to the dish for flavor or added digestive support.

Keep Fresh:
Use fresh seasonal produce! I like to keep a rotating bin of:
Apples, peaches, raspberries, blueberries, figs, squash and zucchini, bell pepper, green beans, avocado, sugar snap peas, celery, asparagus, fennel bulb, sweet potato, potato, carrot, beet, cilantro, parsley, lemon/lime, and leafy greens like kale, collard greens, Bok choy, spinach, chard, dandelion and mustard greens.

In the Garden:

Plant culinary herbs like:

Mint, thyme, rosemary, lavender, jasmine, oregano, lemongrass and dill. There are infinite possibilities here. Learn about what grows native in your region.

An Impeccable Pantry:

Whole Grain Rice (rotate between different types – basmati, jasmine, white, brown, red rice, black volcano rice, etc.)
Quinoa
Split Mung Beans
Red Lentils
Split Peas
Pasta of Choice (whole wheat, rice noodle, etc.)
Nutritional Yeast
Tamari (soy sauce)
Nuts (almond, cashew, walnut, etc.)
Almond Butter
Tahini
Arrowroot Flour
Spelt Flour
Chickpea Flour
Coconut Butter
Medjool Dates
Coconut Milk
Sparkling Water
Goji Berries
Cacao Powder
Seeds like sunflower, pumpkin, flax, and chia
Cashews
Almonds
Whole mineral salts: Himalayan pink salt, black lava salt, sea salt, etc.

Plenty of Good Fats:
Unrefined and as high quality as possible.

Olive Oil
Coconut Oil
Toasted Sesame Oil
Homemade Ghee

Other Options: *Grapeseed Oil, Sunflower Oil, Black Cumin Oil*

Tea and Coffee:

Tulsi Rose Tea
Green Tea
Black Tea (I like decaf, for decaf chai!)
Hibiscus Tea
Egyptian Licorice Tea
Coffee Alternative (Like Cafe Capomo)
Ginger Tea
Peppermint Tea

Sweeteners:

Local Honey
Succanat
Raw Cane Sugar
Maple Syrup
Jaggery

Chilled Essentials for the Refrigerator:

Rotating stock of fresh produce
Sesame seeds
Almond meal
Oat milk (or milk of choice)
Onion (cut in half to absorb toxicity and keep the freshness of the refrigerator!)
Pitted green or kalamata olives
Organic sprouted tofu or tempeh

The Right Tools:

Great Knives: High-quality knives make a world of difference when it comes to chopping vegetables! If you find chopping your hard produce like sweet potatoes and squashes frustrating, I highly recommend investing in a new, high-quality Santoku knife.

A High-Powered Blender: Not just for smoothies but for making great sauces! My favorite brands are Vitamix and Ninja.

Food Processor: Blends and mixes recipes that are too thick for a blender or that need to mix for long periods of time. This is the go-to machine for the *Raw Chocolate Ganache Pie*!

Stainless-Steel Rice Cooker w/ Steam Tray: You can make full meals with just this one appliance at home or at the office. Cook grain in the main compartment and steam vegetables at the same time. See *Quick Office Kitchari Recipe* for a great practical application of the rice cooker. Be sure to avoid the "nonstick" products to keep hazardous toxins out of your kitchen and mouth!

Instant Pot: The Instant Pot is a multifaceted pressure cooker that can be used to cook almost anything! It can sauté, pressure cook, and slow cook. It's electric, can store food airtight, and can be transported easily. It's a great "one pot shop" for individual cooking and large groups. We ran a whole commercial kitchen with Instant Pots and no range!

Common Food Substitutions

Many of these may come in handy for you according to your constitution, health condition, and preferences. The foods listed in the left-column are very common in the modern diet, without question. Many, however, if consumed in excess or improperly can cause or exacerbate many common health ailments. Learning to cook with some of these common substitutions can be fun, flavorful, and beneficial.

Milk	***Almond, Soy, Rice, Hemp, Oat,*** and ***Coconut Milks*** can all be used as a substitution for milk. Each has a unique flavor and thickness that can be used skillfully.
Butter	***Ghee (clarified butter)*** is a flavorful and lighter version of butter that can be substituted for almost all uses of butter. For a non-dairy alternative, use ***Coconut Oil, Olive Oil, or Coconut Butter.***
Cheese	***Nutritional Yeast*** is a great way to make something dairy free but "cheesy." It's a great kitchen staple, with a terrible name. I prefer to call it "hippy flakes." Sprinkle on top as you would parmesan cheese or make sauces mixed with coconut milk, ghee, salt and spices. Great for pasta, risotto, nut cheese, popcorn topping, pesto, etc.

Chicken/ Ground Meat	***Jackfruit*** - This is amazingly delicious, with a "meaty" flavor and texture. Sautéed ***Tofu***. Buy organic hard tofu and sauté with oil (sesame, ghee, etc.) and shoyu (soy sauce) until lightly browned. Add spices or mix into vegetables, legumes, etc. There are also many delicious ***Meat Alternatives*** available, such as Beyond Meat which I recommend only in moderation (because they are processed).
Onion	***Fennel Bulb*** (for texture) – chop and sauté as you would onion. ***Hing (asafoetida)*** – a spice common to Indian cooking resembles the flavor of onion and garlic.
Tomato	***Roasted Red Bell Peppers*** make a great "tomato sauce" that can be used for pasta/pizza sauces and for the base of many traditional recipes. Replace tomato sauce with ***Pesto Sauce*** (recipe included). Make a tomato sauce creamy and delicious by adding ***Coconut Milk*** and ***Nutritional Yeast***, which will lower the tomato and acid content.
Wheat	***Spelt, Rice, Quinoa, Buckwheat, Millet***
Coffee	***Capomo (Maya Nut)*** is an amazing coffee alternative. Or replace coffee with a new ritual of homemade ***Chai*** (there's a great recipe in the recipe section), or ***Herbal Tea*** of your preference.

Peppers/Chili/ Jalapeño	If you need to cut the spice, but still want some pungent flavor, opt for ***Shoshito Pepper***, ***Banana Pepper, Sweet Peppers, Paprika*** or ***Smoky Paprika***.
Black Pepper	Not all black peppers are made equally. The ***Malabar*** variety boasts great health effects, with less penetrating heat. ***White Pepper*** offers a slightly softer effect, while maintaining spice. To eliminate the spicy effect altogether, choose other savory herbs like ***Curry Leaf, Hing, Cumin, Mustard*** and ***Bay Leaf.***
Rice	***Barley, Quinoa, Couscous, Shredded Cauliflower***
Potato	***Rutabaga*** is a great choice, both baked and mashed! Or try other root vegetables to add color and flavor such as ***sweet potato, yam, turnip***, ***beet,*** and ***carrot***. ***Mashed Cauliflower*** is also delicious!
Yogurt	Substitute ***Coconut Yogurt*** or ***Coconut Milk.*** For a sour kick, add a splash of ***Lemon*** or ***Apple Cider Vinegar.***
Alcohol	***Kombucha, Non-Alcoholic Beer,*** and ***Sparkling Cider*** are all classic choices. There are a myriad of great non-alcoholic options that have hit the market just in recent years. Or get creative and create your own ***Mocktails***, using ***Juices, Bitter Tinctures,*** and various ***Sparkling Tonics***. You can even make them medicinal by using tinctures and teas like ***Hibiscus, Rose, Kutki, Moringa, Ashwagandha, Cardamom*** and ***Shatavari***.

White Flour	Nix the empty calories and use whole grain flours like ***Rice, Coconut, Spelt, Almond*** and ***Cassava***. They all have different qualities, tastes, and cooking requirements. Be sure to look them up for proper recipe conversions.

A FEW STAPLE RECIPES

KITCHARI

What is Kitchari?

Kitchari is a classic Ayurvedic dish that consists of a grain, a legume, spices, ghee, and if desired, vegetables. It is considered the "perfect" food because it has an optimal proportion of carbohydrates, protein, and quality fats as well as a tasty mix of digestive spices. This combination creates a healthy and delicious meal that is very easy on the digestive system.

Kitchari can be made using a combination of many different grains (rice, millet, amaranth, barley, etc.) and either lentils (green, yellow, red) or mung beans.

Split and hulled mung beans are optimal for those undergoing Panchakarma, or utilizing this Simple Kitchari Recipe for specific health purposes.

It is a great staple in the diet and can be used for periodic cleanses and during Panchakarma, Ayurveda's Deep-Tissue Detoxification Therapy.

To make 1–2 serving(s):

Ingredients:

2/3 cup Basmati Rice

1/3 cup Sprouted Split Mung Bean (or legume of choice)

1 cup Chopped Vegetables (2–3 from veggie list below)

2 cups Water

1 large Tbsp Ghee

1/2 tsp Turmeric Powder

3/4 tsp Cumin Powder

3/4 tsp Coriander Powder

1/4 tsp Himalayan Pink Salt

1 lemon or lime

You can use a variety of vegetables each time you make kitchari. Choose 2–3 of the following:

Carrot, Sweet Potato, Zucchini, Yellow Squash, Delicata Squash, Pumpkin, Snap Peas, Kale, Spinach, Collard Greens, Mustard Greens, Beets, Turnip, Rutabaga

Cooking Instructions:

Keep a collection of spices, salt, jar of ghee (or oil of choice) as well as a small rice cooker with a steam tray at work or in your kitchen prep area. Stainless steel material is best.

30 minutes before desired mealtime, add rice, legume, turmeric, and water to the basin of the rice cooker. Stir. Place a steam tray on top and add chopped vegetables.

Put the lid on and turn the rice cooker on. Once the cooker finishes cooking, spoon rice mix into a bowl. Add a liberal dollop of ghee, cumin, coriander, and salt (feel free to add more spices to taste). Add vegetables on top. With two forks (or spoons), toss ingredients together thoroughly.

Optional: Squeeze lemon/lime atop, and top it off with cilantro. Enjoy!

Optional Modifications:

- Add more spices, like ginger, black pepper, mustard seed or fenugreek per your taste and constitution.
- Add seaweed
- Stir in nutritional yeast
- Top with a ground seed mixture of chia, flax, sesame, and pumpkin seeds.
- Make vegan by substituting ghee with coconut oil, olive oil or grapeseed oil.
- For wetter kitchari, add more water.

THE BEST ROSEMARY GRAVY

"Gheegan"

This super easy and absolutely scrumptious gravy recipe is one of the all-time favorites of my friends, family and clients! Serve over anything that you'd traditionally pour gravy on top of: mashed potatoes, shepherd's pie, biscuits, dressing, and other traditional Thanksgiving delights.

5 cups water
1 Tbsp of chopped fresh rosemary
1 tsp hing (asafoetida)
1 cup nutritional yeast
2 Tbsp ghee
1/4 cup Tamari
3 Tbsp arrowroot powder
3 Tbsp cold water

Combine water, rosemary, nutritional yeast, ghee, and tahini into a pot and bring to a boil. Boil for 3 minutes. Take off heat.

Mix together arrowroot and cold water. Stir together until a thick milky consistency. Pour slowly into the mixture after it is taken off the heat source and stir immediately.

Modifications:

- Add or replace rosemary with sage, thyme, and/or oregano.
- If you do not have arrowroot powder, cornstarch can be used.

*Note: Not all nutritional yeast is made equally. My favorite brand is Red Star or Bob's Red Mill. If it doesn't make your food taste good, try another brand.

CILANTRO PARSLEY PESTO

This cheese-free rendition of pesto is light and flavorful! Use on pizza, pasta, with spaghetti squash as a dip, or mixed in a quinoa dish. Easily substitute basil, spinach, or other leafy greens for variety!

1 cup fresh parsley
1 cup fresh cilantro
1/3 cup olive oil
1/3 cup raw almonds
1 Tbsp nutritional yeast
3/4 tsp salt
Optional: 1/2 lemon (juice)

Blend all ingredients together in a blender until pasty consistency. Add a dash of water if needed.

ITALIAN RIBOLLITA SOUP

Ribollita Soup is an Italian classic, typically passed down generationally. Learning the family recipe is a serious task and often takes decades to master. This recipe is inspired by a delightful meal around a festive table in Tuscany.

Olive Oil, liberal amounts
2-3 cups water (depending on desired thickness)
2 cans white cannellini beans
1 can of artichoke hearts
1 carrot
2 pieces of celery stalk
1/2 Tbsp fresh, chopped rosemary

1/2 bunch chopped parsley
1/2 zucchini
1 red bell pepper
1/2 Tbsp smokey paprika
1/2 Tbsp hing
1/2 Tbsp Himalayan salt
1/2 Tbsp oregano
1/2 Tbsp thyme
1/2 Tbsp sage
1/4 Tbsp dry ginger
Bread of choice

Preheat oven to 400 degrees. Cut bell pepper in half (long way) and deseed. Place face down on cookie sheet and roast in the oven until charred. Meanwhile, chop vegetables and herbs and sauté in a soup pot liberal amount of olive oil on medium heat. When the bell pepper is done, blend with smoky paprika and 2 Tbsp olive oil to make a creamy paste. Pour onto vegetable mixture and add white beans. Sprinkle salt over the beans. Stir together and simmer on medium heat, stirring regularly. Add 2-3 cups of water or to desired consistency.

Serve over pieces of toasted bread or add a few pieces of bread to sit at the bottom of the soup pot overnight as it's done traditionally.

Top with sprinkled nutritional yeast.

BROTHY SOUP

Brothy soup is a great option for a very light evening meal or even a warm and light start of the day for those who are looking to revamp their digestion and get things "flowing" better. There are many ways to make brothy soup. It can be made with or without vegetables or even legumes, like lentils. A bit of oil or ghee can be added.

One of my favorite versions I call "Iron Water." This is the broth from boiled spinach. Add a bit of salt and some spices (like salt, turmeric, and black pepper) and you have a delicious broth or soup base.

Boil vegetables of choice (such as carrot, spinach, celery, parsley, carrot greens, beet greens, fennel greens, etc.) in a quart of water. Add some digestive spices such as:

- A spoonful of the "Big 3" mix (cumin, coriander & turmeric)
- Ginger and ajwain for a more heating mixture
- Coriander, cilantro, and dill for a more cooling/neutral mixture
- Add garlic and onion if fighting a cold or congestion

For simple broth, strain veggies. Or, leave them to be part of the soup. Add a bit of salt to taste and a teaspoon of oil or ghee for some added lubrication if desired. To add a bit more flavor, try adding a spoonful of nutritional yeast.

Sip first thing in the morning for digestive support or enjoy as a light dinner with an optional piece of flatbread.

ROOT SOUP

"Purple Soup"

As taught in Ayurvedic cooking, this recipe combines all six tastes:

Sweet: *Root vegetables and maple syrup*
Salty: *Himalayan pink Salt*
Astringent: *Turmeric*
Pungent: *Ginger*
Bitter: *Rosemary*
Sour: *Lemon*

Root Soup is great year-round but is particularly delicious in the autumn months!

6 cups water
4 large carrots
3 small–medium sized beets (or 2 large ones)
3 large Jerusalem artichokes (or substitute purple potatoes)
4 generous Tbsp of organic ghee
1/2 tsp turmeric powder
1 ½ tsp dried ginger powder
2 tsp Himalayan pink salt
Juice of 1 lemon
2 Tbsp maple syrup

Topping: 1 handful of fresh rosemary
1 Tbsp coconut oil (or use ghee)
Pinch of salt

Fill the soup pot with water and cook on medium heat. Chop vegetables into 1/2-inch cubes. Add vegetables, ghee, turmeric, and ginger to water. Bring to a boil. Then lower to medium-low heat and cover. Let cook for 20–30 minutes or until veggies are soft enough to easily fork through. Turn heat to low.

Add remaining ingredients. Blend with immersion blender until extra creamy (or leave chunky if you prefer!). If water has evaporated, you may add extra.

For topping, combine all ingredients in a small saucepan. Sauté on medium heat until rosemary begins to lightly brown. Turn off heat.

*Serve soup topped with crisped rosemary. Homemade roti or warmed pita bread on the side goes great!

LEMONGRASS MINT CHAI

Adapted and inspired by Jhankhna Varma.

Makes 3 mugs

~½ - 1 stalk of fresh lemongrass (about 1-2 tsp chopped)

2 black tea or decaf black tea bags

2 peppermint tea bags (or a small handful of freshly chopped mint leaves)

2 cups water

2 cups oat milk (or milk of choice)

~4 spoonfuls of sugar (or sweetener of choice) to liking

Cut string and tag from tea bags if they are present. Combine lemongrass, black tea bags, peppermint tea bags, and water together. If using fresh mint, keep aside (do not add to the water at this time). Bring to a boil and cook on medium heat for 3 minutes. Add oat milk. Cook until the mixture is just about to reach a boil. Turn off heat. If using fresh mint, add now. Strain through fine metal strainer. Add sugar, sucanat or honey to your liking.

This is a great chai for the summer months, and for people with pitta constitutions.

INDIAN CARDAMOM CHAI

This recipe was given by one of our beloved teachers Dr. Bharati Lele, in her home in Pune, India.

Recipe serves 8 cups

Ingredients:

11 Tbsp Loose Leaf Black Tea*

1 Tbsp Freshly Powdered Whole Green Cardamom

1 Tbsp Sucanat (or sweetener of choice)

1 Tbsp Cinnamon Powder

1/2 gallon of Milk, or Oat milk (full fat either way)

1/2 gallon Boiling Water (or a little less depending on how creamy you prefer your chai)

*Harney and Son's Decaf Black Orange Pekoe Loose Leaf Tea, decaffeinated via CO2 process, is our favorite

Cooking Instructions:

Blend fresh cardamom and sugar together in a coffee grinder to a fine powder. Boil the milk and water separately. When both milk and water are at a boil, turn the heat off the milk or reduce to a simmer. Immediately add tea and spices to the boiling water. Boil for just 2 minutes! Pour the tea through a strainer into the milk. Be sure to press the excess tea out of the loose leaves with a ladle. Add sugar to taste in your own chai cup. Drink immediately for maximum flavor.

CACAO DATE SMOOTHIE

This quick and delicious shake is a great morning breakfast ritual as well as an aphrodisiac and effective rejuvenator post-exercise or post-sex. It is full of ojas (vitality). It's like a milkshake that's good for you! It can be a breakfast staple.

Makes 1 serving.

Ingredients:

2 Medjool Dates

1 pinch Cinnamon

1 heaping Tbsp Almond Butter*

1 extra-heaping Tbsp of Cacao Powder

16 oz oat milk or milk of choice

*Alternatively, use a different nut/seed butter such as sunflower butter or peanut butter.

Cooking Instructions:

Blend ingredients together well in a blender. Be sure to de-seed the dates!

Optional Modifications:

- Add a protein or plant collagen powder as an added boost. I'm not a huge fan of packaged "powdered" supplements, but there are a few high quality ones out there, and when used appropriately can be a healthy and effective supplement. I recommend not using a chocolate flavored one. Or, if you do, reduce the cacao in the recipe.
- Substitute cardamom instead of cinnamon.
- Add goji berries for added zinc and other health benefits.
- Replace cacao with carob powder.
- Add half of a banana.

CHOCOLATE GANACHE PIE

This unbaked vegan and gluten-free pie is creamy and divine! It's quick to prepare and is made from whole foods that are healthy and delicious.

Filling

1 ½ cup dark chocolate chips (vegan)
1/2 cup maple syrup
2 large ripe avocados
1 Tbsp vanilla
1/8 tsp salt

Pie Crust

4 cups almonds
10 dates (1.5 cups)
1/4 tsp cinnamon
1/8 tsp ginger
Pinch of nutmeg
Pinch of cardamom
Pinch of sea salt

For filling, combine ingredients together in a food processor and blend until extra creamy. There should be no sign of avocado chunks. Set aside. Separately, combine pie crust ingredients together in your food processor and blend until doughy. Form and press the crust to the bottom of the pie pan. Pour filling and chill for 2–4 hours .

Enjoy!

HOMEMADE GHEE

Clarified Butter

Not all ghee is made the same. The quality of the butter makes a huge difference, as does the quality of the preparation. High quality store-bought ghee is expensive. Fortunately, it's simple and much cheaper to make ghee at home.

Makes one 8 oz. Jar:

Supplies Needed:

1 box of Organic Unsalted Cultured Butter (Organic Valley brand is

good option)

1 Small/Medium Pot

Cheesecloth (quadruple layered)

Small "fine" Metal Strainer or Jar Funnel

16 oz Sanitized Mason Jar

Ladle

Preparation Instructions:

Melt butter on the stove on low-medium heat. Once melted, stir consistently in a clockwise direction. Ghee will go through the following stages as you stir:

1) Melt
2) Milk solids begin to separate
3) Milk solids start coagulating with a dark gold liquid (foam may develop)
4) Solids drop to the bottom and ghee becomes translucent. This is when the ghee is done and ready to be filtered.

Depending on the level of heat, and various other factors, the solids may turn a rusty orange color. This is okay and another sign that the ghee is ready to be filtered.

Place strainer or funnel over jar, and place quadruple-layered cheesecloth on top. Make sure there is absolutely no moisture in the jar. Any moisture in the jar will cause your ghee to mold quickly.

Carefully ladle the ghee into the jar and let it naturally drip through the cheesecloth into the jar. Avoid squeezing the cheesecloth full of solids tightly to optimize ghee drainage, as solids are more likely to escape.

Cover the jar tightly and let it solidify unrefrigerated. Ghee should not be refrigerated.

Traditionally, ghee is made on the full moon and let to moon-bathe overnight outside once it is jarred.

Idea:

Stock up on ghee and make more than one jar at a time! As long as jars are sealed airtight and do not have any moisture inside, ghee does not go bad. Store in a cool, dark place.

CORIANDER TONIC

Traditionally called 'Dhanyaka Hima', this refreshing drink is used in Ayurveda as a tonic for the kidneys and bladder. It is a delicious cooling drink in the summer months to alleviate burning sensations and excessive thirst. The full moon is the best time to prepare this delightful beverage, as the lunar quality enhances the cooling quality!

In a mason jar, or other airtight container, add:
1/2 cup whole coriander seeds
3 cups water
1 Tbsp cane sugar *optional, to taste

Let sit overnight in the refrigerator or outside in the moonlight. In the morning, strain and enjoy.

AVOCADO HONEY FACE MASK

Just like your gut digests what you take in, your skin digests what you put on. The largest organ of the body, the skin protects, digests, and eliminates. Just like our digestion is unique, everyone's skin is different and requires different care. Food based products are fantastic for skin care, as they provide totally natural and effective tools for skin care. If you wouldn't eat it, I generally wouldn't put it on your skin!

This recipe is best for those with dry skin needing moisture and rejuvenation. It's great for aging skin too.

1 ripe avocado
1 tsp raw honey

Splash of milk, almond milk, or oat milk (unsweetened)

*If you'd like to thicken the mixture, add some mung bean powder or ground oats.

Blend all ingredients together to a smooth paste. You can add 1–2 drops of rose or sandalwood essential oil (or powder), if available.

Apply to a freshly cleaned face. Steam first if desired. Leave until mixture starts to dry. Wash with lukewarm water. Spritz with rose water to finish.

OTHER FOOD-BASED SKINCARE TIPS:

Just like every food has different qualities when eaten, each food has unique characteristics when used externally, too.

If you tend to have dry, brittle skin: *You want to use things that are heavy, moisturizing, and oily in nature like almond, milk, avocado, yogurt, and oat (vata-pacifying properties).*

If your skin tends to be congested and oily: *you will want to use foods that are drying, light, and purifying in nature such as neem, mung powder, turmeric, and lemon (kapha-pacifying properties).*

If your skin tends toward redness and inflammation: *Cooling and calming foods are good options, such as rose, coconut, coriander, sandalwood and cucumber (pitta-pacifying properties).*

Thin ***cucumber slices*** are used over the eyes. This is not just for show! Ayurvedically-speaking, it's important to keep the eyes cool (because they are pitta-dominant). Cucumbers are cooling and therapeutic to rest on the eyes.

TURMERIC HONEY WOUND PASTE

Keep this recipe in your forever home "Farmacy!" Turmeric-honey is a classic Ayurvedic remedy to support wound healing. Both substances have numerous medicinal qualities that help to stop bleeding, reduce inflammation, and provide antibacterial properties. I find it cuts healing time by as much as half!

Simple mix together:

1 tsp of honey
1/2 tsp of turmeric

Make into a paste. Apply it directly to a cut or wound and cover with a bandage. The turmeric will stain your skin for a few days, be forewarned!

Keep an eye out for more recipes and healthy cooking tips!

To explore more Ayurvedic recipes, I recommend - *The Everyday Ayurveda Cookbook: A Seasonal Guide to Eating and Living Well* by Kate O'Donnel and Cara Brostrom.

You may also enjoy *The Complete Book of Ayurvedic Home Remedies* by Vasant Lad. This is a great reference that helps turn your kitchen into a natural *farmacy*.

BIBLIOGRAPHY

Albeck-Ripka, Livia. "The 'Great Pacific Garbage Patch' is Ballooning, 87,000 Tons of Plastic and Counting." *New York Times,* March 22, 2018. https://www.nytimes.com/2018/03/22/climate/great-pacific-garbage-patch.html

Areppim. "Nobel Prize Awards by Gender in each Category." Accessed July 29, 2021. https://stats.areppim.com/stats/stats_nobel_sexxcat.htm

Andrews, Gianna. "Plastics in The Ocean affecting Human Health." Accessed September 29, 2012. https://serc.carleton.edu/NAGTWorkshops/health/case_studies/plastics.html

Bischoff, Stephan. C. "'Gut Health': A New Objective in Medicine?" *BMC Medicine* 9, no. 1 (March, 2011): 1-14.

Breit, Sigridr., Aleksandra Kupferberg, A., Gerhard Rogler, and Gregor G., & Hasler., G. (2018). "Vagus Nerve as Modulator of the Brain–Gut Axis in Psychiatric and Inflammatory Disorders." *Frontiers in Psychiatry,* no. 9, (March 2018): 44. https://doi.org/10.3389/fpsyt.2018.00044

Center for Effective Government. *Living in the Shadow of Danger.* Michigan: W.K. Kellogg Foundation, 2016. https://www.foreffectivegov.org/sites/default/files/shadow-of-danger-highrespdf.pdf

Centers for Disease Control and Prevention. "Adult Obesity Prevalence Maps." Accessed June 29, 2021. https://www.cdc.gov/obesity/data/prevalence-maps.html

Cleveland Clinic. "Diaphragmatic Breathing." Accessed June 29, 2021a. https://my.clevelandclinic.org/health/articles/9445-diaphragmatic-breathing

Cleveland Clinic. "Fad Diets." Accessed August 15 2021b. https://my.clevelandclinic.org/health/articles/9476-fad-diets

Cromie, William J. "Pleasure, Pain Activate Same Part of Brain." *The Harvard Gazette,* January 31, 2002. https://news.harvard.edu/gazette/story/2002/01/pleasure-pain-activate-same-part-of-brain/

Davies, Douglas. J., and Michael J. Thate. "Religion and the Individual: Belief, Practice, and Identity." Basel: MDPI-Multidisciplinary Digital Publishing Institute, 2017.

Davis, Shannon N., Sarah Winslow, and David J. Maume. (Eds.). *Gender in the Twenty-First Century: The Stalled Revolution and the Road to Equality*. California: University of California Press, 2017.

Demarinis, Susie. (2020). "Loneliness at Epidemic Levels in America." *Explore,* 16, no. 5(5), (September-October 2020): 278.

Domonoske, Camila. "Students Have 'Dismaying' Inability to Tell Fake News from Real, Study Finds." Accessed May 31, 2021. https://www.npr.org/sections/thetwo-way/2016/11/23/503129818/study-finds-students-have-dismaying-inability-to-tell-fake-news-from-real

Durack, Juliana., and Susan V. Lynch, "The Gut Microbiome: Relationships with Disease and Opportunities for Therapy." *Journal of Experimental Medicine* 216, no. 1 (October 2019): 20-40.

Elder, LeeErica. "Green Thumbs Up." https://www.icphusa.org/wp-content/uploads/2015/01/ICPH_UNCENSORED_3.2_Summer2012_GreenThumbsUp.pdf

Elliott, Carolyn. "Existential Kink: Unmask your Shadow and Embrace your Power (A Method For Getting What You Want By Getting Off On What You Don't)." Newburyport: Weiser Books, 2020.

Farabee, Michael J. "*Laws of Thermodynamics.*" https://www2.estrellamountain.edu/faculty/farabee/biobk/biobookener1.html

Fieldhouse, Paul. *Food and Nutrition: Customs and Culture.* Berlin/Heidelberg: Springer, 2013.

Food and Agriculture Organisation of the United Nations. "Energy-Smart" Food for People and Climate Issue Paper," 2011a. http://www.fao.org/3/i2454e/i2454e.pdf

Food and Agriculture Organization of the United Nations. "Key Facts and Findings," n.d.b. http://www.fao.org/news/story/en/item/197623/icode/

Galen, Karlan-Mason and Rebecca Shi. "The Food Pyramid & How Money Influences USDA Dietary Guidelines. " Accessed May 31, 2021. https://www.greenchoicenow.com/v/food-pyramid-usda-dietary-guidelines

Galvin, Garrett T. *Lone Star Colar: Challenges and Opportunities in Post-blackout Texas.* California: JDSUPRA, 2021. https://www.jdsupra.com/legalnews/lone-star-solar-challenges-and-8224877/

Gardiner, Beth. "The Plastics Pipeline: A Surge of New Production Is on the Way." Accessed September 1, 2021. https://e360.yale.edu/features/the-plastics-pipeline-a-surge-of-new-production-is-on-the-way

Garone, Sarah. "Nutrigenomics Might Be the Future of How You Eat." Accessed July 3, 2021. https://www.healthline.com/health/food-nutrition/nutrigenomics-might-be-the-future-of-how-you-eat

Glader, Eva., Matthew Fraser, M., Gerard Roemers, G., O. Sabag Muñoz, O., Erin Kennedy, and Peter Hirsch., P. (2020, February 14). "What are Macronutrients and Micronutrients." Accessed April 20, 2021. https://www.getsmarter.com/blog/market-trends/what-are-macronutrients-and-micronutrients/

Gotter, Ana. "Gallbladder Diet." Accessed August 27, 2021. https://www.healthline.com/health/gallbladder-diet

Gut Microbiota for Health by ESNM. "Gut Microbiota Info." Accessed February 2, 2021. https://www.gutmicrobiotaforhealth.com/about-gut-microbiota-info/

Hanania, Nicola A., Sidney Braman, Sandra G. Adams, Ruth Adewuya, Arzu Ari, JoAnn Brooks, Donald A. Mahler, Jill A. Ohar, Jay Peters, and Shahin Sanjar. "The Role of Inhalation Delivery Devices in COPD: Perspectives of Patients and Health Care Providers."

Chronic Obstructive Pulmonary Diseases: Journal of the COPD Foundation 5, no. 2 (April 2018): 111. https://doi.org/110.15326/jcopdf.5.2.2017.0168.

Harvard Health Publishing. "Understanding the Stress Response." Accessed May 17, 2021. https://www.health.harvard.edu/staying-healthy/understanding-the-stress-response

Hilliard, Jena. "Study Reveals Gen Zas the Loneliest Generation in America." May 22, 2021. https://www.addictioncenter.com/news/2019/08/gen-z-loneliest-generation/

Hooke, Andy. "Cheese: A Brief History And The Origins Of Why Americans Can't Get Enough." Accessed May 31, 2021. https://switch4good.org/too-much-cheese

SHAPES THROUGH HISTORY

International Energy Agency. "Petrochemicals Set to be the Largest Driver of World Oil Demand, Latest IEA Analysis Finds." Accessed January 16, 2021a. https://www.iea.org/news/petrochemicals-set-to-be-the-largest-driver-of-world-oil-demand-latest-iea-analysis-finds

International Renewable Energy Agency. "Majority of New Renewables Undercut Cheapest Fossil Fuel on Cost."Accessed June 19, 2021b. https://www.irena.org/newsroom/pressreleases/2021/Jun/Majority-of-New-Renewables-Undercut-Cheapest-Fossil-Fuel-on-Cost

Johns Hopkins Medicine. "Diaphragmatic Breathing" Accessed June 2, 2021. https://www.hopkinsallchildrens.org/Services/Anesthesiology/

Pain-Management/Complementary-Pain-Therapies/Diaphragmatic-Breathing

Klenerman, Leslie. *Human Anatomy: A Very Short Introduction*. Oxford: OUP Oxford, 2015.

Kotchoubey, Boris. "Human Consciousness: Where Is It From and What Is It For." *Frontiers in Psychology* 9 (April, 2018): 567.

Lesser, Elizabeth. *Cassandra Speaks: When Women are the Storytellers, The Human Story Changes*. New York: HarperCollins.

Lumen. *Functions of the Autonomic Nervous System.* Accessed July 12, 2021. https://courses.lumenlearning.com/boundless-ap/chapter/functions-of-the-autonomic-nervous-system/

Lotter, Eugene. *Your Gut is The Cornerstone of Your Immune System*. Accessed July 12, 2021. https://www.news24.com/health24/medical/flu/preventing-flu/your-gut-is-the-cornerstone-of-your-immune-system-20160318

Mayer, Emeran. *The Mind-Gut Connection: How The Hidden Conversation Within Our Bodies Impacts Our Mood, Our Choices, and Our Overall Health*. New York: HarperCollins, 2018.

McKay, Pamela, Patrick Fielding, Eve Gallop-Evans, Georgina W. Hall, Jonathan Lambert, Mike Leach, Teresa Marafioti, Christopher McNamara, and British Committee for Standards in Haematology. "Guidelines for the investigation and management of nodular lymphocyte predominant Hodgkin lymphoma."

British Journal of Haematology 172, no. 1 (2016): 32-43. https://doi.org/10.1111/bjh.13842.

Molnar, Charles and Jane Gair. *Concepts of Biology.* Victoria: BCcampus, 2015.

Moore, Erin. *How to Stop Eating Junk Food: 10 Tips to Control your Cravings.* Accessed January 23, 2021. https://www.healthline.com/health/food-nutrition/how-to-stop-eating-junk-food

National Health Council. "About Chronic Diseases." Accessed February 14, 2021. https://nationalhealthcouncil.org/wp-content/uploads/2019/12/AboutChronicDisease.pdf

Nunez, Christina. "Deforestation Explained." Accessed March 23, 2021. https://www.nationalgeographic.com/environment/article/deforestation

Pandey, M. M., Subha Rastogi, and A. K. S. Rawat."Indian Traditional Ayurvedic System of Medicine and Nutritional Supplementation." *Evidence-Based Complementary and Alternative Medicine*, 2013. https://doi.org/10.1155/2013/376327

Perel, Esther. *Mating in Captivity: Reconciling the Erotic and the Domestic.* New York: HarperCollins, 2006. https://www.goodreads.com/book/show/27485.Mating_in_Captivity

Physiopedia. "Vagus Nerve." Accessed July 2, 2021. https://www.physio-pedia.com/Vagus_Nerve

Pisharodi, Sanjay. "Acharya Vagbhata's Astanga Hrdayam: The Essence of Ayurveda (Vol. 1)." CreateSpace Independent Publishing, 2016.

Porges, Stephen W. and Deb Dana. *Clinical Applications of the Polyvagal Theory: The Emergence of Polyvagal-Informed Therapies (Norton Series on Interpersonal Neurobiology)*. New York: WW Norton & Company, 2018.

Rain-Tree Publishers. "About the Rainforest." Accessed August 15, 2021. https://rain-tree.com/facts.htm

Reuters. "A Plateful of Plastic." Accessed 20 May, 2021. https://graphics.reuters.com/ENVIRONMENT-PLASTIC/0100B4TF2MQ/index.html

Richards, Joni, Laurel Dicus, Sarah Drexler, Anna-Claire Gibson, and Caleigh Lentz. "Case Study of the Dove for Real Beauty Campaign." https://en.calameo.com/books/00337511237b2e84ea999

Roser, Max. and Hannah Ritchie. "Hunger and Undernourishment." Accessed May 25, 2021. https://ourworldindata.org/hunger-and-undernourishment#too-little-height-for-age-stunting

Sapulpa Times. "Nature Knows Best: What is The Vagus Nerve?!" Accessed 3 March, 2021. https://sapulpatimes.com/nature-knows-best-what-is-the-vagus-nerve/

Savage, Jennifer, Jennifer Orlet Fisher, and Leann L. Birch. . "Parental Influence on Eating Behavior: Conception to Adolescence." *The Journal of Law, Medicine & Ethics* 35, no.1 (Spring 2007): 22-34. https://doi.

org/10.1111/j.1748-720X.2007.00111.x

Seymour, Tom. "Everything you Need to Know about the Vagus Nerve." Accessed July 21, 2021. https://www.medicalnewstoday.com/articles/318128

Shea, John M. "The Digestive System." New York: Gareth Stevens Publishing LLLP, 2012.

Skoczylas, Erin. "Foodprint: How Our Diet Affects the Carbon Footprint." Accessed January 16, 2021.

Statista. "Total Sugar Consumption Worldwide from 2009/2010 to 2021 (in Million Metric Tons)." Accessed August 17, 2021. https://www.statista.com/statistics/249681/total-consumption-of-sugar-worldwide/#:~:text=The%20global%20consumption%20of%20sugar,more%20widely%20available%20than%20eve

The Washington Post. "You're Literally Eating Microplastics. How You Can Cut Down Exposure to Them." Accessed March 31, 2021. https://www.washingtonpost.com/health/youre-literally-eating-microplastics-how-you-can-cut-down-exposure-to-them/2019/10/04/22ebdfb6-e17a-11e9-8dc8-498eabc129a0_story.html

Venniro, Marco, Marco Zhang, Daniele Caprioli, Jennifer K. Hoots, Sam A. Golden, Conor Heins, Marisela Morales, David H. Epstein, and Yavin Shaham. "Volitional Social Interaction Prevents Drug Addiction in Rat Models." *Nature Neuroscience* 21, no. 11 (October 2018): 1520-1529.

Wanjek, Christopher. (2012, July 27). "Your Diet Affects Your Grandchildren's DNA, Scientists Say." Accessed January 29, 2021. https://www.livescience.com/21902-diet-epigenetics-grandchildren.html

Waxman, Adam J, Suparna Clasen, Wei-Ting Hwang, Alfred Garfall, Dan T. Vogl, Joseph Carver, Rupal O'Quinn, Adam D. Cohen, Edward A. Stadtmauer, Bonnie Ky, and Brendan M. Weiss. "Carfilzomib-Associated Cardiovascular Adverse Events: A Systematic Review and Meta-Analysis." *JAMA Oncology* 4, no. 3 (2018): e174519-e174519. https://doi.org/10.1001/jamaoncol.2017.4519.

Wikipedia. "Tonga." Accessed March 2, 2021. https://en.wikipedia.org/wiki/Tonga

World Wildlife Fund. "Climate Change in the Amazon." Accessed March 21, 2021. https://wwf.panda.org/discover/knowledge_hub/where_we_work/amazon/amazon_threats/climate_change_amazon/?

Wren, Gavin. "The Ritual of Coffee." Accessed February 7, 2021. https://brainfoodstudio.com/writing/ritual-of-coffee/

Wu, Hsin-Jung, and Eric Wu. "The Role of Gut Microbiota in Immune Homeostasis and Autoimmunity." *Gut Microbes* 3, no.1(January 2012): 4-14.

Yehuda, Rachel., and Amy Lehrner. "Intergenerational Transmission of Trauma Effects: Putative Role of Epigenetic Mechanisms." *World Psychiatry* 17, no. 3 (September 2018): 243-257.

Book Jacket Design:
Rocco J. Santoro
info@thesantorogroup.com

Cover Floral Arrangement:
Barbara Santora
Barbara's Bloomers

Cover Photo:
John Hendricks

CPSIA information can be obtained
at www.ICGtesting.com
Printed in the USA
BVHW070315301121
622779BV00009B/573

9 781637 921883